Essentials of

Pharmaceutical Chemistry

Essentials of
Pharmaceutical Chemistry

Second edition

Donald Cairns
BSc, PhD, MRPharmS, CChem, MRSC

Associate Head of School of Pharmacy
The Robert Gordon University
Aberdeen, UK

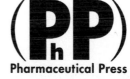

London • Chicago   **Pharmaceutical Press**

Published by the Pharmaceutical Press
Publications division of the Royal Pharmaceutical Society of Great Britain

1 Lambeth High Street, London SE1 7JN, UK
100 South Atkinson Road, Suite 206, Grayslake, IL 60030-7820, USA

(**P.P**) logo is a trade mark of Pharmaceutical Press

First edition published 2000
Second edition published 2003

Text design by Barker/Hilsdon, Lyme Regis, Dorset
Typeset by Mathematical Composition Setters Ltd, Salisbury, Wiltshire
Printed in Great Britain by TJ International, Padstow, Cornwall

ISBN 0 85369 570 9   *1003515366*

A catalogue record for this book is available from the British Library

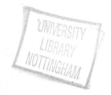

For Elaine, Andrew and Mairi

Contents

Preface to second edition

It is nearly three years since the first edition of *Essentials of Pharmaceutical Chemistry* was published. In that time a number of changes have been made to undergraduate courses in pharmacy and pharmaceutical science. A university degree evolves with time as a result of internal factors such as university reorganisation and external factors such as accreditation by professional bodies. This new edition has been written in response to some of these changes.

New chapters have been included on physicochemical properties of drugs, stereochemistry and drug metabolism, and existing chapters on acids and bases, partition coefficient and biopharmacy have been updated and extended.

I am grateful to all the readers of the first edition who commented on the book. I have tried, wherever possible, to include their suggestions in this new edition, even though some were contradictory.

Thanks are also due to the staff at The Pharmaceutical Press for all their assistance and patience, especially Lorraine Parry, for the coffee and muffins.

Donald Cairns
February, 2003

Preface to first edition

This book is about pharmaceutical chemistry, that is, the chemistry of drugs. When the man in the street hears the term 'drugs' or if asked to name a drug, he will most probably come up with the name of a drug of abuse, e.g. heroin, morphine, cocaine, amphetamine. This book is not about these compounds (although a lot of what this book is about does apply to these compounds); rather, this book is concerned with drugs in their widest possible meaning. It is important to remember that the vast majority of drug use in the world is beneficial to the recipient. In the USA the public is told to 'say no to drugs' yet the American public spends almost $75 billion a year on 'over the counter' and prescription medicines.

A good general definition of a drug is 'a chemical substance which, when taken, affects some physiological function within the body'. This definition applies whether it be aspirin acting to remove the pain of a headache or penicillin destroying the bacteria causing an infection. If we pursue this definition, it leads to the conclusion that the term 'drugs' includes everything from simple gaseous elements such as oxygen (used for resuscitation), with a molecular mass of 32 Da, right through to large protein molecules with relative molecular masses of several thousand, such as Factor VIII, the blood clotting factor used to treat haemophiliac patients. Indeed, with the advent of gene targeting and gene-specific agents, the possible size range for drugs increases to relative molecular masses of a million or more. However, most drugs are simple organic molecules which are usually water soluble and usually either a weak acid or a weak base. This is important because acids and bases can ionise, i.e. they can donate protons, or hydrogen ions, to their environment (in the case of acids) or accept protons from their surroundings (in the case of bases). The process of ionisation changes the physicochemical properties of the compound dramatically, particularly its solubility in aqueous solution.

The first chapter of the book is, therefore, concerned with the chemistry of acids and bases, while the second deals with the effects of ionisation on the solubility and partitioning properties of drugs.

The third and fourth chapters deal with the volumetric and spectroscopic analysis of drugs and medicines.

The subsequent chapters of the book deal with stability of drug molecules and prediction of shelf-life of medicines.

Each chapter ends with some tutorial examples of the types of calculation described within the chapter. There are also some problems to allow the reader to test if they have understood the material. Answers are supplied at the end of the book. These problems are all taken from recent end of term or module examinations in pharmacy or pharmaceutical science.

Donald Cairns
April, 2000

Acknowledgements

This book could not have been completed without the help of a great many people. I am very grateful to my colleagues, past and present for their advice and encouragement and particularly, for allowing me to assimilate their good practice (with or without their knowledge!). This book would be poorer without their efforts. Special thanks must go to Paul Hambleton who read and commented on my first drafts and who not only allowed me to use a great many of his examination questions but also provided most of the answers!

I am grateful to Paul Weller, Linda Horrell, Helen Bond and all the staff at the Pharmaceutical Press for keeping me on track when diversions threatened and giving helpful advice about indexes, content pages, etc.

Finally, I must thank my wife, Elaine, who looked after the weans while I bashed the keyboard upstairs.

About the author

Donald Cairns obtained a Bachelor of Science degree in pharmacy from the University of Strathclyde in 1980 and after a pre-registration year spent in hospital pharmacy, he returned to Strathclyde to undertake a PhD on the synthesis and properties of benzylimidazolines. Following a year as a post-doctoral research fellow in the department of pharmacy at Sunderland Polytechnic (now the University of Sunderland), Dr Cairns moved to Leicester Polytechnic (now De Montfort University) where he held a five-year lectureship in Pharmacy. In 1992 Dr Cairns was appointed senior lecturer in medicinal chemistry in Sunderland School of Pharmacy and has recently been appointed Associate Head of the School of Pharmacy at Aberdeen. He has been an external examiner in Liverpool and Aberdeen Schools of Pharmacy and has authored over 50 peer-reviewed research papers.

His research interests include the design and synthesis of selective anticancer agents, the molecular modelling of drug/DNA interactions and the design of prodrugs for the treatment of nephropathic cystinosis.

Donald Cairns is a member of the Royal Pharmaceutical Society of Great Britain (RPSGB), the Royal Society of Chemistry and the RPSGB's Academy of Pharmaceutical Scientists.

To travel hopefully is a better thing than to arrive, and the true success is to labour.

Robert Louis Stevenson, 1850–1894

1

Chemistry of acids and bases

Chemistry is the defining science of pharmacy. Everything about a drug, its synthesis, the determination of its purity, the formulation into a medicine, the dose given, the absorption and distribution around the body, the molecular interaction of drug with its receptor, the metabolism of the drug and, finally, the elimination of drug from the body requires a thorough and comprehensive understanding of the chemical structure of the drug and how this chemical structure influences the properties and behaviour of the drug in the body. For these reasons, chemistry is the most important of all the scientific disciplines contributing to the understanding of drugs and their actions in the body. A good understanding of the chemistry of drugs will allow the study of advanced topics such as drug design and medicinal chemistry, molecular pharmacology and novel drug delivery systems that usually occur in the later stages of a pharmacy or pharmaceutical science degree.

As stated in the preface, most drugs are small organic molecules that behave in solution as either weak acids or weak bases. In order to understand and appreciate these compounds a study must be made of simple acid–base theory.

In 1887, the Swedish chemist Arrhenius suggested that solutions that conduct electricity (so-called electrolytes) do so because they dissociate into charged species called ions. Positively charged ions (or *cations*) migrate towards the negative terminal, or cathode, while negatively charged ions (or *anions*) migrate towards the positive terminal, or anode. It is this movement of ions that allows the passage of electric current through the solution.

Compounds of this type may be classified as strong electrolytes, which dissociate almost completely into ions in solution, or as weak electrolytes, which only dissociate to a small extent in solution. Since strong electrolytes are almost completely dissociated in solution, measurement of the equilibrium constant for their dissociation is very difficult. For weak electrolytes, however, the dissociation can be expressed by the law of mass action in terms of the equilibrium constant.

Considering the reaction

$$A + B \rightleftharpoons C + D$$

the equilibrium constant (K) for the reaction is given by the product of the concentrations of the reaction products divided by the product of the concentrations of the reactants, or

$$K = \frac{[C] \times [D]}{[A] \times [B]}$$

Clearly, if the equilibrium lies to the right-hand (or products) side, the numerator in the above expression will be greater than the denominator, and K will be greater than 1. Conversely, if the reaction does not proceed to completion, $[A] \times [B]$ will be larger than $[C] \times [D]$ and K will be less than 1.

Strictly speaking, the law of mass action states that 'the rate of a chemical reaction is proportional to the active masses of the reacting substances', but for dilute solutions active mass may be replaced by concentration, which is much easier to measure.

The law of mass action can be applied to the dissociation of water, a weak electrolyte widely used as a solvent in biological and pharmaceutical systems:

$$H_2O \rightleftharpoons H^+ + OH^-$$

The equilibrium constant for this reaction is given by

$$K = \frac{[H^+] \times [OH^-]}{[H_2O]}$$

In pure water, and in dilute aqueous solutions, the concentration of molecular water, $[H_2O]$ is so large as to be considered constant (approximately 55.5 M), so the above expression simplifies to

$$K_w = [H^+] \times [OH^-] \tag{1.1}$$

and K_w is called the *ionic product of water*. The value of this equilibrium varies with temperature but is usually quoted as 1×10^{-14} at 25 °C. The units of K_w are mole litre^{-1} × mole litre^{-1}, or mole^2 litre^{-2} (also sometimes written as mole^2 dm^{-6} where 1 dm^3 = 1 litre).

Since, in pure water, $[H^+] = [OH^-]$, the hydrogen ion concentration in water is given by the square root of K_w, which is 1×10^{-7} mole litre^{-1}.

Solutions in which the hydrogen ion concentration is greater than 10^{-7} M are called acidic, while solutions with a concentration of hydrogen ions of less than 10^{-7} mole litre^{-1} are referred to as alkaline.

The range of hydrogen ion concentrations encountered in chemistry is very large, so it is convenient to adopt the pH notation first developed by another Scandinavian chemist, Sørensen. He defined pH as 'the negative logarithm (to the base 10) of the hydrogen ion concentration'. or

$$pH = -\log_{10}[H^+] = \log_{10}\frac{1}{[H^+]}$$

Use of the pH notation allows all degrees of acidity and alkalinity normally encountered in chemistry to be expressed on a scale from 0 to 14, corresponding to the concentrations of H^+ ions contained in the solution. Solutions with a pH < 7 are considered acidic, solutions with a pH > 7 are alkaline, while a solution with a pH = 7 is neutral.

It should be noted that a sample of water will often give a pH reading of less than 7, particularly if the sample has been left in an open beaker. This is due to carbon dioxide present in the atmosphere dissolving in the water to give carbonic acid (H_2CO_3), which dissociates to release H^+ ions.

Dissociation of weak acids and bases

Acids are compounds that ionise to release hydrogen ions, or protons, to their surroundings. Bases are compounds that can accept hydrogen ions. This is called the Brønsted–Lowry definition of acids and bases. There are other ways of explaining acidity and basicity, but the Brønsted–Lowry theory works most of the time, and will be used throughout this book.

The dissociation of a weak acid is usually represented as follows:

$$HA \rightleftharpoons H^+ + A^-$$

However, this suggests that protons exist free in solution like little tennis balls bouncing around chemical reactions. The reality is that protons are *solvated* in solution, that is they go around attached to a solvent molecule. Since the most common solvent in pharmaceutical and biological systems is water, the ionisation of a weak acid is better represented as

$$HA + H_2O \rightleftharpoons H_3O^+ + A^-$$

where H_3O^+ is a *hydroxonium* ion, and the ionisation of a base can be represented as

$$B + H_2O \rightleftharpoons BH^+ + OH^-$$

It is important to notice that water appears in these equations as both a proton acceptor and a proton donor. This is an example of the *amphoteric* or *amphiprotic* nature of water. Although the ionisation of acids and bases in water is best described using the equations above, it is convenient to disregard the water when deriving useful expressions and relationships.

Consider any weak acid, HA, which dissociates as shown below:

$$HA \rightleftharpoons H^+ + A^-$$

The equilibrium constant for this reaction is given, as before, by

$$K = \frac{[H^+] \times [A^-]}{[HA]}$$

In the case of an acid dissociation, the equilibrium constant for the reaction is termed K_a, and is called the ionisation or dissociation constant. The above equation can now be rewritten as

$$K_a = \frac{[H^+] \times [A^-]}{[HA]}$$

For exact work, the concentration term must be replaced by the thermodynamic activity of the ion, but for dilute solutions concentration may be used.

K_a is a constant for a given compound at a given temperature. Clearly, the farther the above equilibrium lies to the right-hand side, the more completely will the acid ionise and the greater will be the value of K_a. To put it more simply, the greater the value of K_a, the stronger is the acid.

Using the equation above, it is possible to derive an expression for the strength of acid solutions. If the acid, HA, ionises to α moles of H^+ ions and α moles of OH^- ions, where α is the fraction of the acid that is ionised, then the number of moles of undissociated acid is given by $(1 - \alpha)$. This acid solution can now be prepared with c moles of acid in 1 litre (or 1 dm^3), which will yield αc moles of H^+ and αc moles of A^-. Hence,

$$HA \rightleftharpoons H^+ + A^-$$

$$(1 - \alpha)c \rightleftharpoons \alpha c + \alpha c$$

$$K_a = \frac{\alpha c \times \alpha c}{(1 - \alpha)c}$$

$$K_a = \frac{\alpha^2 c^2}{(1 - \alpha)c}$$

$$K_a = \frac{\alpha^2 c}{(1 - \alpha)}$$

For weak electrolytes, α is very small and may be neglected so $(1 - \alpha)$ is approximately = 1. The simplified expression may now be written as

$$K_a = \alpha^2 c$$

where c is the concentration, in moles per litre, and α is the degree of ionisation of the acid. Then

$$\alpha = \sqrt{\left(\frac{K_a}{c}\right)}$$

The pH of the solution can now be determined:

$$[H^+] = \alpha c$$

Therefore,

$$[H^+] = c \sqrt{\left(\frac{K_a}{c}\right)} = \sqrt{(K_a c)}$$

Taking logarithms,

$$\log[H^+] = \tfrac{1}{2} \log K_a + \tfrac{1}{2} \log c$$

Multiplying throughout by -1 gives

$$-\log[H^+] = -\tfrac{1}{2} \log K_a - \tfrac{1}{2} \log c$$

Therefore,

$$pH = \tfrac{1}{2}pK_a - \tfrac{1}{2} \log c \qquad\qquad (1.2)$$

Equation (1.2) applies to the ionisation of weak acids, but a similar expression can be derived for weak bases. The equation for the ionisation of a weak base may be expressed as

$$B + H_2O \rightleftharpoons BH^+ + OH^-$$

$$(1 - a)c \rightleftharpoons ac + ac$$

where B is the base and BH^+ is termed the *conjugate acid* of the base. The equilibrium constant for this reaction is written as

$$K_b = \frac{[BH^+] \times [OH^-]}{[B]}$$

$$K_b = \frac{a^2 c}{(1 - a)}$$

As before α is very small and can be neglected, so $(1 - \alpha)$ is approximately $= 1$.

$$\alpha^2 = \frac{K_b}{c}$$

$$\alpha = \sqrt{\left(\frac{K_b}{c}\right)}$$

From above,

$$[OH^-] = c\alpha$$

Therefore,

$$[OH^-] = c \sqrt{\left(\frac{K_b}{c}\right)} = \sqrt{(K_b c)}$$

However,

$$[OH^-] = \frac{K_w}{[H^+]}$$

Therefore,

$$\frac{K_w}{[H^+]} = \sqrt{(K_b c)}$$

and

$$[H^+] = \frac{K_w}{\sqrt{(K_b c)}}$$

Taking logarithms,

$$\log[H^+] = \log K_w - \tfrac{1}{2}\log K_b - \tfrac{1}{2}\log c$$

or

$$\mathbf{pH} = \mathbf{p}K_w - \tfrac{1}{2}\mathbf{p}K_b + \tfrac{1}{2}\log c \tag{1.3}$$

Equations (1.2) and (1.3) are extremely useful because they allow the pH of solutions of weak acids and bases to be calculated if the concentrations and dissociation constant are known.

How strong an acid is depends on how many hydrogen ions are released when the acid ionises, and this depends on the degree of ionisation, α, for any given concentration. As stated above, K_a, the equilibrium constant for the dissociation of the acid, gives a measure of how far the ionisation equilibrium lies to the right-hand, or products, side. As can be seen from equation (1.3), a similar expression, K_b, gives a measure of basic strength and, as with K_a, the higher the numerical value of K_b, the stronger is the base.

It is often useful and convenient to express the strengths of acids and bases using the same term, pK_a, and this can be done by considering the equilibria that exist between an acid and its conjugate base. A weak acid (HA) and its conjugate base (A^-) are related as follows:

$$HA \rightleftharpoons H^+ + A^-$$
$$A^- + H_2O \rightleftharpoons HA + OH^-$$

From the equations above,

$$K_a = \frac{[H^+] \times [A^-]}{[HA]} \quad \text{and} \quad K_b = \frac{[HA] \times [OH^-]}{[A^-]}$$

Then

$$K_a \times K_b = \frac{[H^+] \times [A^-]}{[HA]} \times \frac{[HA] \times [OH^-]}{[A^-]}$$

Cancelling similar terms gives

$$K_a \times K_b = [H^+] \times [OH^-]$$

which can be rewritten as

$$K_a \times K_b = K_w = 1 \times 10^{-14} \qquad (1.4)$$

That is, the acid dissociation constant and the base dissociation constant are related through the ionic product of water.

Equation (1.4) is a very important relationship since it allows the calculation of K_b or K_a if the other is known. It also follows that the strengths of acids and their conjugate bases are related through K_w. This means that a strong acid must have a weak conjugate base and, similarly, a weak acid must have a strong conjugate base. A moment's thought will confirm that this must, indeed, be true. Acids and their conjugate bases are related by equilibria, which can be thought of as giant seesaws. If one partner of the pair is very strong and heavy, the other will be weak and light. The same relationship applies to acid–conjugate base equilibria.

This relationship also allows chemists to be lazy and express the strengths of acids and bases in terms of the dissociation constant for the acid. This is particularly true when we consider the term pK_a.

In a similar manner to pH, the pK_a of an acid is defined as the negative logarithm (to the base 10) of the dissociation constant, K_a, i.e.

$$pK_a = -\log_{10} K_a$$

This terminology allows chemists to talk loosely about the pK_a of acids and bases, when what they really mean is the pK_a of acids and the conjugate acids of bases. It is incorrect to say 'the pK_a of a primary amine is between 9 and 10', although the usage is widespread. It is more accurate to say 'the pK_a of the conjugate acid of a primary amine is between 9 and 10'. This is just another example of lecturers saying one thing and meaning another.

Another source of confusion concerning strengths of acids arises with K_a and pK_a. The term K_a is the dissociation constant for the ionisation of an acid, and hence the larger the value of K_a, the stronger is the acid (since the equilibrium constant lies farther to the right-hand side). pK_a is the negative logarithm of K_a, and is used commonly because K_a values for organic acids are very small and hard to remember (typically 10^{-5}). It follows that since pK_a is the *negative* logarithm of K_a, the smaller the value of pK_a the stronger is the acid.

Consider the two carboxylic acids below:

Acetic acid, CH_3COOH, $pK_a = 4.7$

Chloroacetic acid, $ClCH_2COOH$, $pK_a = 2.7$

In answer to the question, 'which acid is the stronger?', clearly it is chloroacetic, since its pK_a is smaller. A student of organic chemistry could even suggest that the reason is due to increased stabilisation of the anion formed on ionisation by the electronegative chlorine atom. If the question is asked 'how much stronger is chloroacetic than acetic?', then all sorts of interesting answers appear, ranging from 'twice as strong' to a 'million times as strong'. The answer, obvious to anyone who is familiar with logarithms, is that chloroacetic is 100 times stronger than acetic acid. This is because the difference in pK_a is two units on a log scale, and the antilog of 2 to the base 10 is 100. It is important for students (and graduates!) to appreciate that pH and pK_a are *logarithmic* relationships and that a K value corresponding to a pK_a of 2.7 is not really close to a K value corresponding to a pK_a of 4.7.

Equation (1.4) can be rewritten into a logarithmic form by taking the negative logarithm of both sides, to give

$$pK_a + pK_b = pK_w = 14 \tag{1.5}$$

Hydrolysis of salts

When a salt is dissolved in water, the compound dissociates completely to give solvated anions and cations. This breaking of bonds by the action of water is called *hydrolysis* and the salt is said to be *hydrolysed*. The pH of the resulting solution depends on whether the salt was formed from reaction of strong or weak acids and bases and there are four possible combinations.

For example, if the salt results from reaction between a strong acid and a strong base (e.g. NaCl), then the resulting solution will be neutral, and NaCl is termed a neutral salt. Of the two ions produced, Na^+ and Cl^-, only the Cl^- reacts with water:

$$Cl^- + H_2O \rightleftharpoons HCl + OH^-$$

This reaction does not occur to any great extent since the Cl^- is the conjugate base of a strong acid, namely HCl. The Cl^- is therefore a very weak conjugate base and its reaction with water can be neglected.

If the salt results from reaction between a strong acid and a weak base (e.g. the reaction of ammonia and hydrogen chloride to give ammonium chloride)

$$HCl + NH_3 \rightleftharpoons NH_4^+ + Cl^-$$

then the resulting salt solution will be acidic by hydrolysis and the pH of an aqueous solution of the salt will be less than 7.

This can be demonstrated by considering the reactions that occur when ammonium chloride is hydrolysed. The salt dissociates completely to give hydrated ammonium ions and hydrated chloride ions. The Cl^- ion is not very reactive towards water, but the ammonium ions react with water to give ammonium hydroxide. This is because NH_4^+ is the conjugate acid of the weak base NH_3, and must therefore be quite strong. The NH_4^+ reacts with water as follows to produce H_3O^+ ions:

$$NH_4^+Cl^- \rightleftharpoons NH_4^+ + Cl^-$$
$$NH_4^+ + H_2O \rightleftharpoons NH_3 + H_3O^+$$

An increase in the concentration of H_3O^+ ions results in a fall in pH, and an acidic solution.

The pH of this solution can be calculated by using the equation derived for a weak acid, equation (1.2) above:

$$pH = \tfrac{1}{2}pK_a - \tfrac{1}{2}\log c$$

If the salt results from the reaction of a strong base and weak acid (e.g. sodium acetate from reaction of sodium hydroxide and acetic acid), then the solution formed on hydrolysis will be basic, i.e.

$$NaOH + CH_3COOH \rightleftharpoons CH_3COO^-Na^+ + H_2O$$
$$CH_3COO^-Na^+ + H_2O \rightleftharpoons CH_3COOH + OH^- + Na^+$$

Na^+ does not react with water to any great extent, but CH_3COO^- is the conjugate base of the weak acid CH_3COOH and is therefore strong enough to react with water to produce OH^- ions.

The increase in concentration of OH^- gives a basic solution, the pH of which can be calculated from the equation for the pH of weak bases, equation (1.3).

$$pH = pK_w - \tfrac{1}{2}pK_b + \tfrac{1}{2}\log c$$

The final scenario involves a salt formed between a weak acid and weak base (e.g. ammonium acetate, $NH_4^+CH_3COO^-$). The H^+ and OH^- ions formed by hydrolysis of ammonium acetate occur in roughly equal concentrations, which will yield a neutral salt.

These relationships can be summarised as follows:

> *Strong acid + Strong base → Neutral salt*
> *Strong acid + Weak base → Acidic salt*
> *Weak acid + Strong base → Basic salt*
> *Weak acid + Weak base → Neutral salt*

and do seem to follow a type of logic. Using the seesaw analogy for equilibria again, if both partners are strong or both are weak, then the seesaw balances, and the solution formed by hydrolysis is neutral. If either partner is strong (or heavy!) then the seesaw tilts to that side to give an acidic or basic solution. This analogy is not precise, but it may help the desperate student remember the pH values of hydrolysed salt solutions.

Buffer solutions

A buffer solution is a solution that resists changes in pH. If acid is added then, within reason, the pH does not fall; if base is added, the pH does not rise. Buffers are usually composed of a mixture of weak acids or weak bases and their salts and function best at a pH equal to the pK_a of the acid or base involved in the buffer. The equation that predicts the behaviour of buffers is known as the Henderson–Hasselbalch equation, and is another vitally important equation worth committing to memory. It is derived as follows, by considering a weak acid that ionises in solution:

$$\mathbf{HA \rightleftharpoons H^+ + A^-}$$

The equilibrium constant for this ionisation is given by

$$K_a = \frac{[H^+] \times [A^-]}{[HA]}$$

Taking logarithms of both sides and separating the hydrogen ion term gives

$$\log K_a = \log[H^+] + \log \frac{[A^-]}{[HA]}$$

Multiplication throughout by -1 gives

$$-\log K_a = -\log[H^+] - \log \frac{[A^-]}{[HA]}$$

or

$$pK_a = pH - \log \frac{[A^-]}{[HA]}$$

which rearranges to give

$$pH = pK_a + \log \frac{[A^-]}{[HA]}$$

Since the acid in question is weak, the number of A^- ions derived from dissociation of the acid itself is very small compared to the number derived from the fully ionised salt. This means that $[A^-]$ is approximately equal to total concentration [SALT]; and similarly [HA], since the acid is weak and predominantly unionised, is approximately equal to the total acid concentration [ACID]. The equation can now be rewritten as

$$pH = pK_a + \log \frac{[SALT]}{[ACID]} \tag{1.6}$$

The Henderson–Hasselbalch equation can also be derived from consideration of the ionisation of a weak base, B, which ionises in aqueous solution as follows:

$$B + H_2O \rightleftharpoons BH^+ + OH^-$$

In this case the [SALT] term can be replaced by the concentration of the conjugate acid of the weak base, $[BH^+]$, which, in effect, yields the same equation.

An example of a buffer is a mixture of acetic acid and sodium acetate, which will ionise as follows:

$$CH_3COOH \rightleftharpoons CH_3COO^- + H^+$$
$$CH_3COO^-Na^+ \rightleftharpoons CH_3COO^- + Na^+$$

Since the acetic acid only ionises to a small extent, there will be a high concentration of undissociated acid (shown in bold) or, to put it another way, the equilibrium for the reaction will lie predominantly to the left-hand side. Sodium acetate is a salt and will ionise completely to give high concentrations of CH_3COO^- and Na^+ (shown in bold).

If H^+ ions are now added to the buffer solution, they will react with the high concentration of CH_3COO^- present to give undissociated acetic acid. Acetic acid is a weak acid and only dissociates to a small extent, so the pH of the solution does not decrease. In effect, a strong acid such as H^+ is mopped up by the buffer to produce a weak acid, acetic acid, which is not sufficiently acidic to lower the pH.

$$H^+ + CH_3COO^- \rightleftharpoons CH_3COOH$$

Similarly, if OH^- ions are added to the buffer system, the OH^- will react with the high concentration of free acetic acid present to give water and acetate ions:

$$OH^- + CH_3COOH \rightleftharpoons H_2O + CH_3COO^-$$

Neither water nor acetate is sufficiently basic to make the solution alkaline, so the pH of the buffer solution will not increase.

The high concentration of sodium ions has little or no effect on the pH of the solution since when these ions react with water they do so to produce equal numbers of H^+ and OH^- ions as shown below:

$$Na^+ + H_2O \rightleftharpoons Na^+OH^- + H^+$$

and

$$Na^+OH^- \rightleftharpoons Na^+ + OH^-$$

Buffers can also be composed of weak bases and their salts; examples include ammonia buffer, used to control the pH of compleximetric titrations (see Chapter 6) and the common biological buffer TRIS (or tris(hydroxymethylaminomethane), $C_4H_{11}NO_3$), used to control the pH of protein solutions.

Buffer capacity

Buffer solutions work best at controlling pH at pH values roughly equal to the pK_a of the component acid or base, i.e. when the [SALT] is equal to the [ACID]. This can be shown by calculating the ability of the buffer to resist changes in pH, which is the *buffer capacity*.

The buffer capacity is defined as the number of moles per litre of strong monobasic acid or base required to produce an increase or decrease of one pH unit in the solution. When the concentrations of salt and acid are equal, the log term in the Henderson–Hasselbalch equation becomes the logarithm of 1, which equals 0. To move the pH of the buffer solution by one unit of pH will require the Henderson–Hasselbalch equation to become

$$pH = pK_a + \log \frac{10}{1}$$

It will require addition of more acid or base to move the pH by one unit from the point where $pH = pK_a$ than at any other given value of the ratio. This can be neatly illustrated by the following example.

Suppose a buffer consists of 0.1 M CH_3COOH and 0.1 M $CH_3COO^-Na^+$, the pH of this buffer solution will be 4.7 (since the log term in the Henderson–Hasselbalch equation cancels). Now, if 10 mL of 1 M NaOH is added to this buffer, what will be the new pH?

Clearly, the 10 mL of NaOH will ionise completely (strong alkali) and some of the 0.1 M acetic acid will have to convert to acetate anion to compensate. The new pH will be

$$pH = pK_a + \log \frac{[SALT]}{[ACID]}$$

$$pH = 4.7 + \log \frac{(0.1 + 0.01)}{(0.1 - 0.01)}$$

$$pH = 4.7 + \log \frac{0.11}{0.09}$$

$$pH = 4.79$$

The addition of 10 mL of 1 M alkali has only increased the pH of the buffer by a small amount. By way of comparison, if 10 mL of 1 M NaOH were added to 1 litre of pure water, the pH of the solution would increase from a pH of 7 to a value of approximately 12 (since pOH for 0.01 M NaOH = 2 and pH + pOH = 14, the pH of the solution = 12).

The buffer capacity (β) for this buffer is given by

$$\beta = \frac{\text{No. of moles of NaOH added}}{\text{Change in pH observed}}$$

$$\beta = \frac{0.01}{(4.79 - 4.7)}$$

$$\beta = \frac{0.01}{0.09}$$

$$\beta = 0.11$$

Since buffer solutions work best at a pH equal to the pK_a of the acid or base of which they are composed, consideration of the pK_a will determine choice of buffer for a given situation. The pK_a of acetic acid is 4.7, and therefore an acetic acid–acetate buffer would be useful for buffering a solution to a pH of approximately 5. Similarly, an alkaline buffer can be obtained by using ammonia solution, which will buffer to a pH of approximately 10 (pK_a of ammonia = 9.25).

If a buffer is required to control the pH of a neutral solution, use is made of the second ionisation of phosphoric acid. Phosphoric acid is a tribasic acid, which requires three equivalents of NaOH as follows:

$$H_3PO_4 + NaOH \rightleftharpoons Na^+H_2PO_4^- + H_2O \qquad pK_a = 2.12$$
$$Na^+H_2PO_4^- + NaOH \rightleftharpoons (Na^+)_2HPO_4^{2-} + H_2O \qquad pK_a = 7.21$$
$$(Na^+)_2HPO_4^{2-} + NaOH \rightleftharpoons (Na^+)_3PO_4^{3-} + H_2O \qquad pK_a = 12.67$$

A mixture of sodium dihydrogen phosphate, $Na^+H_2PO_4^-$ and disodium hydrogen phosphate, $(Na^+)_2HPO_4^{2-}$ will function as a buffer and control the pH to a value of approximately 7.0. In this example, the species with the greater number of available hydrogens functions as the acid, i.e. $Na^+H_2PO_4^-$, while the $(Na^+)_2HPO_4^{2-}$ functions as the salt.

The choice of buffer to use in a given situation therefore depends on the pK_a of the acid or base involved. As a general rule, buffer solutions work well within plus or minus one pH unit of the pK_a. Beyond these values, the buffer capacity is too small to allow effective buffer action.

Biological buffers

The human body contains many buffer systems, which control the pH of body compartments and fluids very effectively. Blood plasma is maintained at a pH of 7.4 by the action of three main buffer systems: first, dissolved carbon dioxide, which gives carbonic acid (H_2CO_3) in solution, and its sodium salt (usually sodium bicarbonate, $NaHCO_3$). This is responsible for most of the buffering capacity. The other two buffers are dihydrogen phosphate ($H_2PO_4^-$), also with its sodium salt, and protein macromolecules. Proteins are polymers composed of repeating units called amino acids. These amino acids (as their name suggests) are compounds containing NH_2 and COOH groups in the same molecule and have the general formula shown in Figure 1.1.

Proteins are composed of about 20 different amino acids, which are connected to each other by *peptide bonds* formed between one amino acid and its neighbour. The side-chain of the amino acid may be

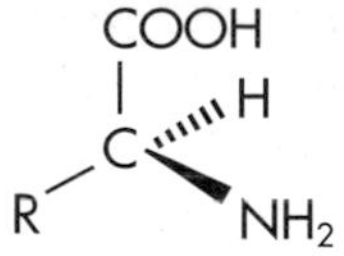

$$COOH$$
$$|$$
$$R-C\overset{\text{\textbackslash\textbackslash\textbackslash}H}{\underset{NH_2}{\diagdown}}$$

Figure 1.1 The general formula of amino acids.

acidic (as in the case of glutamic and aspartic acids), basic (as in the case of arginine and lysine) or neutral (as in alanine). A protein, which may be composed of hundreds of amino acids, is therefore a polyelectrolyte whose properties depend on the balance of acidic and basic groups on the side-chains. Generally, most proteins act as weak acids and form buffers with their sodium salts. Compounds like amino acids, which are capable of acting as both acids and bases, are known as *amphoteric*, or sometimes, *amphiphilic*. In solution, free amino acids usually do not exist in the molecular form shown in Figure 1.1, but instead both the amino and carboxyl groups ionise to form an internal salt as shown in Figure 1.2.

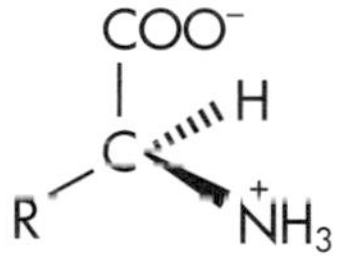

$$COO^-$$
$$|$$
$$R-C\overset{\text{\textbackslash\textbackslash\textbackslash}H}{\underset{\overset{+}{N}H_3}{\diagdown}}$$

Figure 1.2 The structure of a zwitterion.

These internal salts are known by the German word *zwitterion* (German for 'dipolar ion'), and formation of the zwitterion makes the amino acid very polar and therefore very soluble in water. If acid is added to the zwitterion, the ionised COO^- group will accept a proton to give undissociated COOH. The overall charge on the amino acid will now be positive, due to the NH_3^+. Similarly, if base is added to the zwitterion, the NH_3^+ (which is really the conjugate acid of NH_2) will function as an acid and donate its proton to the base. The overall charge on the amino acid will now be negative, due to the ionised COO^-. Amino acids are, therefore, ionised at all values of pH. They are positively charged at low pH, negatively charged at high pH and zwitterionic at neutral pH. The fact that amino acids are ionised at all values of pH and are zwitterionic at neutral pH has profound implications for the oral absorption and bioavailability of amino acids from the diet. The body has to resort to specialised uptake mechanisms to ensure that sufficient levels of these

essential nutrients are absorbed (see Chapter 2). The ionisation of the
simplest amino acid, glycine, is represented in Figure 1.3.

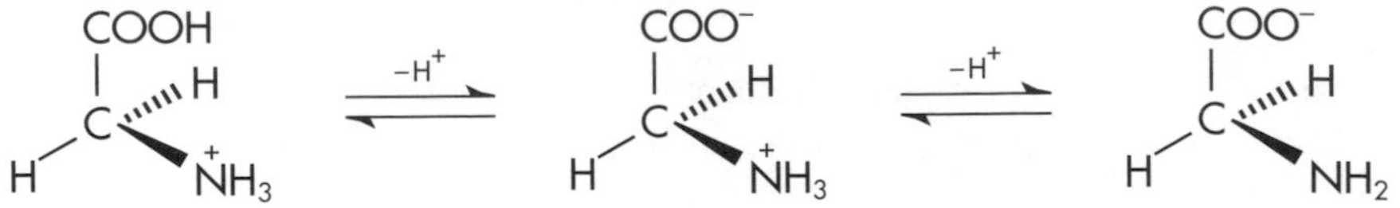

Figure 1.3 The ionisation of glycine.

If the pH of the protein or amino acid solution is adjusted so that
the number of ionised COO^- groups is equal to the number of ionised
NH_3^+ groups, then that value of pH equals pI, the *isoelectric point* of the
protein or amino acid. This point corresponds to the minimum solubility of the protein, and the point at which migration of the protein in an
electric field is slowest (as in the technique of *electrophoresis*, which is
used to separate mixtures of proteins according to their overall electrical
charge). The isoelectric point for an amino acid may be easily calculated
if the pK_a values for the NH_3^+ and COO^- are known (e.g. by titration).
For a simple amino acid, such as glycine, the pI is simply the average of
the two pK_a values. For more complex amino acids, such as glutamic
acid or arginine, which have ionisable groups in the side-chains, the pI
is given by averaging the two pK_a values that lie on either side of the
zwitterion. This is true no matter how many times an amino acid or
peptide ionises. For an amino acid with one acidic group on the side-
chain, there are three distinct ionisations and hence three distinct pK_a
values. Fully protonated aspartic acid ionises as shown in Figure 1.4.
The first group to ionise (and hence the strongest acid) is the
COOH group on the α carbon. This gives pK_{a1}. The second proton is
lost from the side-chain COOH to give pK_{a2}. Finally, the NH_3^+ on the α
carbon ionises to give pK_{a3}. There is, of course, only one pI, which is
given by the average of the two pK_a values on either side of the zwitterion, i.e. $\frac{1}{2}(pK_{a1} + pK_{a2})$. The other commonly occurring amino acid
with an acidic side-chain is glutamic acid. This compound is probably
best known as its monosodium salt (monosodium glutamate or MSG).
This salt is added to foods (especially oriental food) to enhance the
flavour and impart a 'meat-like' taste to the food. Interestingly, both the
D enantiomer of glutamic acid and the naturally occurring L form are
used as food additives. Use of the non-natural D isomer may account for
some of the adverse reactions experienced by consumers of MSG in
food.

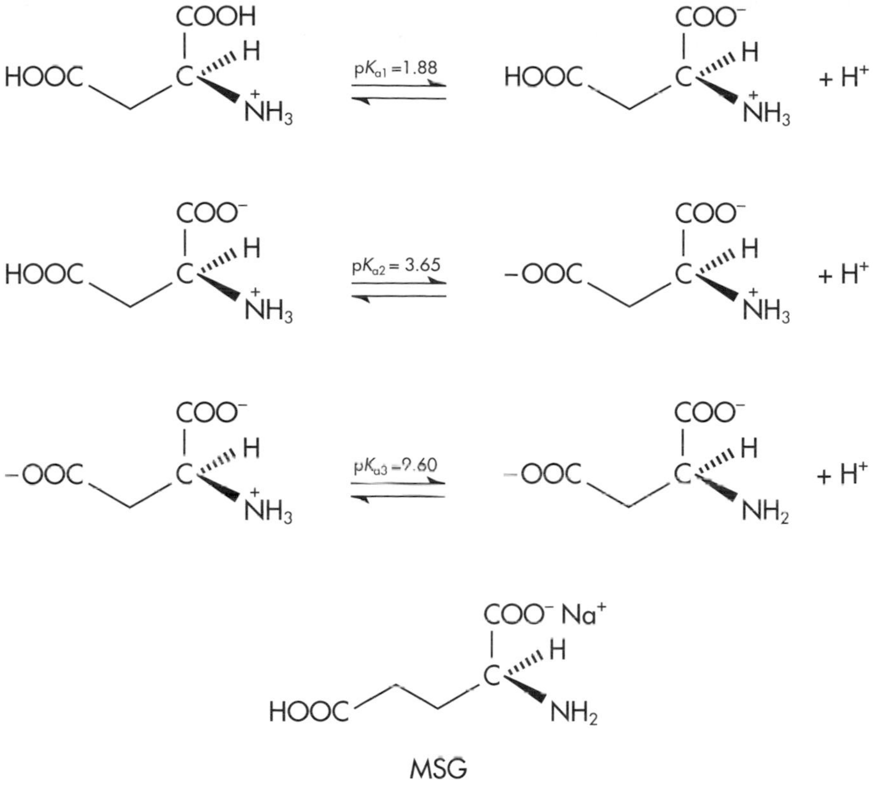

Figure 1.4 The ionisation of aspartic acid and structure of MSG.

Ionisation of drugs

When a weakly acidic or basic drug is administered to the body, the drug will ionise to a greater or lesser extent depending on its pK_a and the pH of the body fluid in which it is dissolved. The pH of the body varies widely, but the most important biological solution is the blood, which, as stated above, normally has a pH of 7.4. An equation can be derived that will predict the extent to which the drug ionises, and, as is often the case, the starting point for the derivation is the Henderson–Hasselbalch equation.

$$pH = pK_a + \log \frac{[\text{SALT}]}{[\text{ACID}]} \qquad (1.6)$$

$$pH = pK_a + \log \frac{[A^-]}{[HA]}$$

Rearranging,

$$pK_a - pH = \log \frac{[HA]}{[A^-]}$$

and, therefore,

$$[HA] = [A^-] \times \text{antilog } (pK_a - pH)$$

The fraction of the total drug that is ionised is given by

$$\frac{[A^-]}{[HA] + [A^-]}$$

so that the fraction ionised is

$$\frac{[A^-]}{[A^-] \times \text{antilog } (pK_a - pH) + [A^-]}$$

which simplifies to

$$\text{Fraction ionised} = \frac{1}{1 + \text{antilog } (pK_a - pH)} \tag{1.7}$$

Equation (1.7) applies to drugs that are weak acids and allows the fraction of the total dose that is ionised to be calculated for any pH if the pK_a of the drug is known. The equation is sometimes written as the percentage ionised, which is simply given by

$$\% \text{ Ionised} = \frac{100}{1 + \text{antilog } (pK_a - pH)} \tag{1.8}$$

A similar expression can be derived for drugs that are weak bases, to give equations (1.9) and (1.10) below.

$$\text{Fraction ionised for basic drug} = \frac{1}{1 + \text{antilog } (pH - pK_a)} \tag{1.9}$$

and

$$\% \text{ Ionised for basic drug} = \frac{100}{1 + \text{antilog } (pH - pK_a)} \tag{1.10}$$

pK_a values of drug molecules

Most compounds used in medicine are either weak acids or weak bases (and quite a few are both!). This means that the range of possible pK_a values encountered in drug molecules is huge. It is important to

Table 1.1 pK$_a$ *values of some common drugs*

Drug	pK$_a$ value
Acidic drugs	
Aspirin	3.5
Paracetamol	9.5
Phenobarbital	7.4 (first ionisation)
Basic drugs	
Cocaine	8.6
Diazepam	3.3
Diphenhydramine	9.0
Amphoteric drugs	
Morphine	8.0 (amine), 9.9 (phenol)
Adrenaline (epinephrine)	8.7 (amine), 10.2, 12.0 (phenols)

remember that the value of the pK$_a$ for a drug tells you *absolutely nothing* about whether the compound is an acid or base. The pK$_a$ value is simply the negative logarithm of the dissociation constant and can, within reason, have any value. This contrasts with the pH notation, where a pH value < 7 means that the solution is acidic and a pH value > 7 means that it is alkaline.

It would be quite wrong to say that because one particular acid has a pK$_a$ of 3, then all compounds with a pK$_a$ of 3 must be acids. Many weak bases have pK$_a$ values of 2 to 4. Similarly, while a basic drug like cocaine has a pK$_a$ of 9.5, this does not mean that all compounds with a pK$_a$ greater than 7 are bases. Indeed, phenols, which are weak acids, mostly have pK$_a$ value of approximately 10. *Only a thorough understanding of chemical structure and a knowledge of the functional groups that confer acidity or basicity on a molecule will allow the correct prediction of the acidic or basic nature of a molecule.* To illustrate this, Table 1.1 lists some common acidic and basic drugs with their pK$_a$ values.

pH indicators

In Chapter 6, the long-suffering reader will encounter volumetric analyses. This technique involves the accurate addition of volumes of solution in order to determine the purity of drugs and raw materials. The end point of many of these titrations can be determined by the colour change of an indicator. The indicators used in pH titrations are themselves weak acids or bases that change colour depending on whether they are ionised or not. The best indicators change colour sharply at a given pH and tables of indicators and their pH range are available. The ionisation of indicators is determined by the Henderson–Hasselbalch equation, where pK_a refers to the negative logarithm of the acid dissociation constant of the indicator, and [SALT] and [ACID] refer to the concentrations of the ionised and unionised forms of the indicator, respectively. If the indicator is a weak base, the Henderson–Hasselbalch equation has to be rewritten as

$$pH = pK_a + \log \frac{[BASE]}{[ACID]}$$

since the salt term is really the conjugate acid of the weak base.

The choice of an indicator for a titration can be made by predicting the pH at the end point of the titration. This is done accurately by working out the proportion of each species at the end of the titration, using the equations above, and determining also the pH due to hydrolysis of any salts present; it may be estimated (and a lot of miserable algebra avoided) as follows.

If the pH of the end point solution is equal to the pK_a of the acid or conjugate acid involved, then there will be equal concentrations of the ionised and unionised forms of the compound present. This is because if $pH = pK_a$ then the log term in the Henderson–Hasselbalch equation is 1 and [unionised] = [ionised]. If the pH of the solution is increased to one unit above the pK_a of the acid (or one unit below the pK_a of the conjugate acid), then the percentage of the compound ionised increases to about 90%. If the pH increases to two units above the pK_a (or two units below for a base), the percentage ionised increases to 99%, since both pH and pK_a are logarithmic relationships, and so on to 99.9%, 99.99% etc. This approximate 'rule of thumb' is summarised below.

For weak acids:

$pH = pK_a$	compound is approximately 50% ionised
$pH = pK_a + 1$	compound is approximately 90% ionised
$pH = pK_a + 2$	compound is approximately 99% ionised
$pH = pK_a + 3$	compound is approximately 99.9% ionised
$pH = pK_a + 4$	compound is approximately 99.99% ionised

For weak bases:

$pH = pK_a$	compound is approximately 50% ionised
$pH = pK_a - 1$	compound is approximately 90% ionised

$pH = pK_a - 2$	compound is approximately 99% ionised
$pH = pK_a - 3$	compound is approximately 99.9% ionised
$pH = pK_a - 4$	compound is approximately 99.99% ionised

This relationship is hugely important and well worth committing to memory. It will reappear many times in this book, in many different guises, and will allow the reader to impress colleagues (particularly medical colleagues) with their uncanny understanding of pH and ionisation of drugs.

In the case of predicting the pH at the end point of titrations, most acid–base reactions are considered over when the ratio of ionised form to unionised form is 1000 to 1, i.e. when

$$pH = pK_a + \log \frac{(99.9)}{(0.1)}$$

From the rules above, this point is reached when the pH of the solution is three units above the pK_a of the acid (or three units below the pK_a of the conjugate acid of the base), and this allows an appropriate indicator to be chosen.

For example, if the acid being titrated has a pK_a of 4.7, then the end point pH will be 4.7 + 3 = 7.7, and an indicator that changes colour between pH 7.0 and 8.0 should be chosen. Similarly, for a base with a pK_a of 8.5, the end point pH will be 8.5 − 3 = 5.5, and an indicator with a pH range of 5.0–6.0 should be used. The pH range of many common indicators is shown in Chapter 6 (p. 135).

Tutorial examples

> *1   Ephedrine is a naturally occurring drug useful in the treatment of asthma. Its structure is shown in Figure 1.5.*
> *(a)   Classify ephedrine as acidic, basic or neutral.*
> *(b)   Using your answer to part (a) as a guide suggest a simple way in which the water solubility of the drug could be increased.*

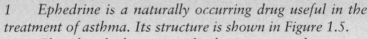

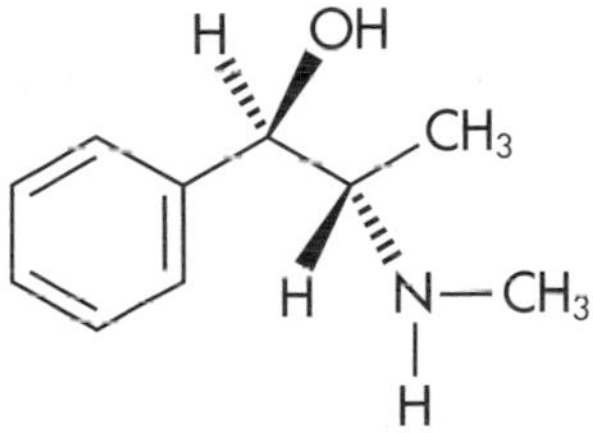

Figure 1.5   The structure of ephedrine, $pK_a = 9.6$.

1(a) Ephedrine is an alkaloid produced by Ephedra (the *Ma huang* plant). It was widely used for the relief of bronchospasm associated with an attack of asthma. The drug has been super-seded in recent years by safer, more effective bronchodilators such as salbutamol and terbutaline. The diastereoisomer of ephedrine, pseudoephedrine, is widely used in cough mixtures as a decongestant. Ephedrine is a secondary amine and, because the lone pair of electrons on the nitrogen can react with H$^+$ ions, is basic in solution (Figure 1.6).

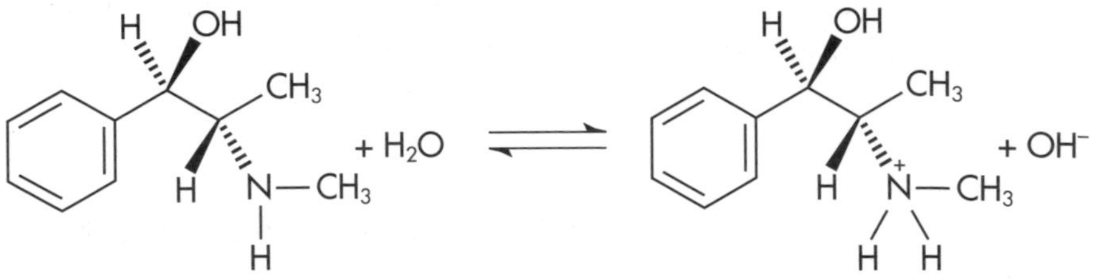

Figure 1.6 Reaction of ephedrine with water.

(b) The water solubility of the drug could be increased by forming a salt with a mineral acid such as hydrochloric acid to give ephedrine hydrochloride (Figure 1.7).

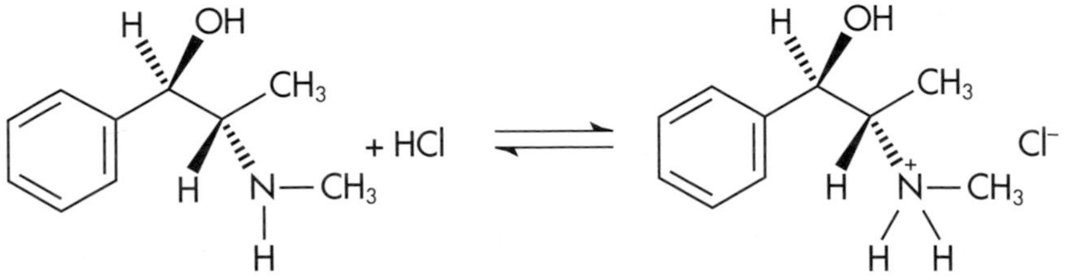

Figure 1.7 Reaction of ephedrine with hydrochloric acid.

This salt will be acidic by partial hydrolysis (salt of a weak base and a strong acid). The pH of the salt solution is given by equation (1.2).

$$pH = \tfrac{1}{2}pK_a - \tfrac{1}{2}\log c$$

If 1 M HCl is reacted with 1 M ephedrine, the resulting concentration of ephedrine hydrochloride will be 0.5 M; therefore,

$$pH = \tfrac{1}{2}pK_a - \tfrac{1}{2}\log c$$
$$= \tfrac{1}{2}(9.6) - \tfrac{1}{2}\log (0.5)$$
$$= 4.8 - (-0.15)$$
$$pH = 4.95$$

which, as predicted, is on the acidic side of neutral. Incidentally, note that the concentration of ephedrine hydrochloride formed above is not 1 M, which may be supposed initially. One mole of ephedrine does give one mole of salt, but the volume of the solution will double when the HCl is added, so the concentration will be halved.

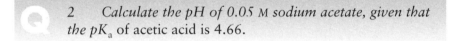

2   *Calculate the pH of 0.05 M sodium acetate, given that the pK_a of acetic acid is 4.66.*

2   Since sodium acetate is the salt of a strong base and a weak acid, it will be basic by partial hydrolysis. We can therefore use equation (1.3) for weak bases to calculate the answer.

$$pH = pK_w - \tfrac{1}{2}(pK_b - \log c)$$
$$pH = 14 - \tfrac{1}{2}(14 - 4.66) + \tfrac{1}{2}\log 0.05$$
$$pH = 14 - 4.67 + (-0.65)$$
$$pH = 8.68$$

3   *Calculate the concentration of acetic acid to be added to a 0.1 M solution of sodium acetate to give a buffer of pH 5 (pK_a of acetic acid = 4.66).*

3   Acetic acid is a weak acid, so its degree of ionisation is very small and the contribution to the total concentration of acetate anions from ionisation of the acid can be ignored. The total salt concentration is therefore 0.1 M from the fully ionised sodium acetate.

Using the Henderson–Hasselbalch equation (equation 1.6),

$$pH = pK_a + \log \frac{[SALT]}{[ACID]}$$

$$5.0 = 4.66 + \log \frac{0.1}{[ACID]}$$

$$0.34 = \log \frac{0.1}{[ACID]}$$

$$2.188 = \frac{0.1}{[ACID]}$$

$$[ACID] = 0.046 \text{ M}$$

4 Weak acids and bases are often formulated as their salts to make them more water soluble. The ionised salts, however, do not cross biological membranes very well. Calculate the percentage of a dose of pentobarbital that will be ionised at plasma pH (7.4). The structure of pentobarbital is shown in Figure 1.8.

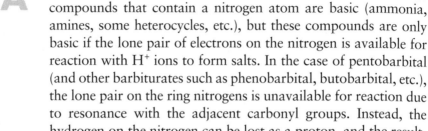

Figure 1.8 The structure of pentobarbital, $pK_a = 8.0$.

4   Pentobarbital is a barbiturate and is a weak acid. Normally, compounds that contain a nitrogen atom are basic (ammonia, amines, some heterocycles, etc.), but these compounds are only basic if the lone pair of electrons on the nitrogen is available for reaction with H^+ ions to form salts. In the case of pentobarbital (and other barbiturates such as phenobarbital, butobarbital, etc.), the lone pair on the ring nitrogens is unavailable for reaction due to resonance with the adjacent carbonyl groups. Instead, the hydrogen on the nitrogen can be lost as a proton, and the resulting negative charge delocalised around the molecule as shown in Figure 1.9.

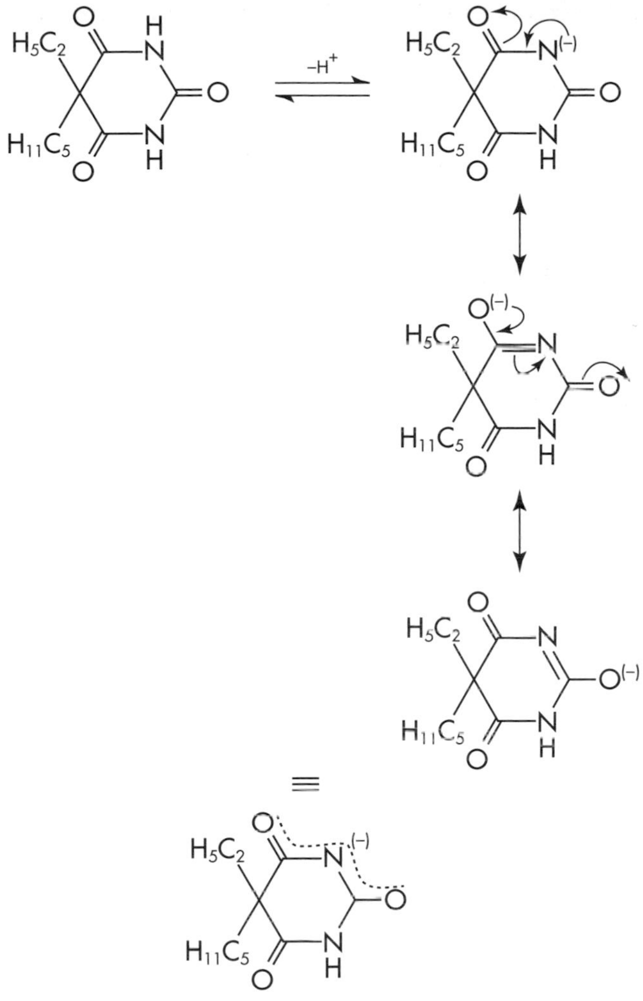

Figure 1.9   Resonance forms of the pentobarbital anion.

This *resonance-stabilised anion* allows barbiturates to function as weak acids, and sodium salts may be formed to increase the water solubility of the drug and allow parenteral administration.

To calculate the percentage ionised, use can be made of equations of the type

$$\% \text{ Ionised} = \frac{100}{1 + \text{antilog} (pK_a - pH)}$$

which is easily derived from the Henderson–Hasselbalch equation and will work for weak acids if the pK_a is known. However, in this case an expression can easily be derived from first principles. If we let x = % ionised,

$$pH = pK_a + \log \frac{[SALT]}{[ACID]}$$

$$7.4 = 8.0 + \log \frac{x}{(100 - x)}$$

$$-0.6 = \log \frac{x}{(100 - x)}$$

$$\frac{x}{(100 - x)} = \text{antilog } (-0.6) = 0.251$$

$$x = 0.251(100 - x)$$

$$x = 25.1 - 0.251x$$

$$x = \frac{25.1}{1.251} = 20.1$$

% Ionised at pH 7.4 = 20.1%

% Unionised at pH 7.4 = 79.9%

Problems

Q1.1   (a)   Ethanolamine $(HOCH_2CH_2NH_2$, relative molecular mass = 61.08) has a pK_a of 9.4. Explain what this term means.

       (b)   Explain why ethanolamine is freely soluble in water, and why the resulting solution is basic.

       (c)   Calculate the pH of a 1% w/v solution of ethanolamine.

       (d)   A solution of pH 9.0 is required that will resist changes in pH on the addition of small amounts of strong acid or strong base. Indicate briefly a possible composition of such a solution, and show how pH changes are resisted.

Q1.2   (a)   What do you understand by the term pK_a? Explain how this value can be used to indicate the strength of a base.

(b) The base ephedrine has a pK_a value of 9.6. Calculate the theoretical end point pH when a 0.1 M solution of ephedrine is titrated with 0.1 M HCl.

(c) Acetic acid (CH_3COOH) has a pK_a value of 4.76. How might you prepare an acetate buffer with a pH of 5.0, containing 0.1 mol L^{-1} of the acid?

(d) Calculate the buffer capacity of the solution described above.

Q1.3   Describe the ionisation or ionisations that occur when fully protonated lysine (Figure 1.10) is subjected to increasing pH. What is the dominant structure present at the isoelectric point?

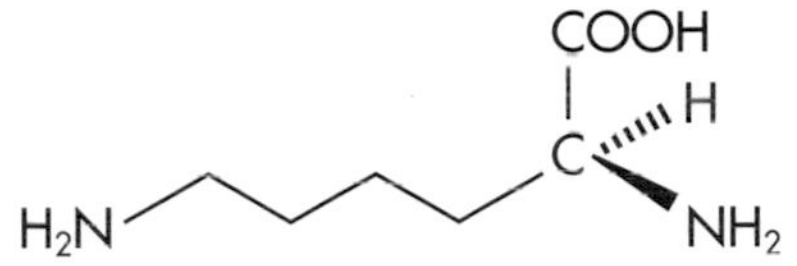

Figure 1.10   The structure of lysine.

(Answers to problems can be found on pp. 213–215.)

2

Partition coefficient and biopharmacy

When a substance (or *solute*) is added to a pair of immiscible solvents, it distributes itself between the two solvents according to its affinity for each phase. A polar compound (e.g. a sugar, amino acid or ionised drug) will tend to favour the aqueous or polar phase, whereas a non-polar compound (e.g. an unionised drug) will favour the non-aqueous or organic phase. The added substance distributes itself between the two immiscible solvents according to the partition law, which states that 'a given substance, at a given temperature, will partition itself between two immiscible solvents in a constant ratio of concentrations'. This constant ratio is called the *partition coefficient* of the substance, and may be expressed mathematically as

$$P = \frac{[\text{organic}]}{[\text{aqueous}]} \tag{2.1}$$

where P is the partition coefficient of the substance; [organic] is the concentration of substance in the organic, or oil phase; and [aqueous] is the concentration of substance in the water phase.

As an example, consider the distribution of 100 mg of a drug between 50 mL of an organic solvent (e.g. ether, chloroform or octanol) and 50 mL of water. The drug is added to the two immiscible solvents in a separating funnel and allowed to equilibrate. When the organic layer is analysed, it is found to contain 66.7 mg of compound. From these data the partition coefficient and the percentage of the drug extracted into the organic layer can be calculated (see Figure 2.1).

The mass of drug in the water phase = 100 − 66.7 mg = 33.3 mg; the concentration of drug in the organic phase = 66.7/50 = 1.33 mg mL^{-1}, and the concentration of drug in the water phase = 33.3/50 = 0.67 mg mL^{-1}. Therefore, the partition coefficient is given by

$$\frac{[\text{organic}]}{[\text{aqueous}]} = \frac{1.33 \text{ mg mL}^{-1}}{0.67 \text{ mg mL}^{-1}} = 2$$

The partition coefficient is a ratio of concentrations, so the units cancel and P has no units.

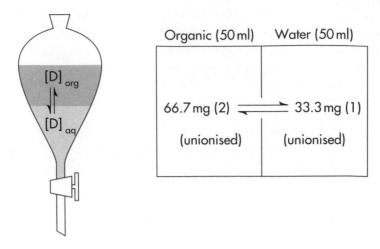

Organic (50 ml)   Water (50 ml)

$[D]_{org}$

$[D]_{aq}$

66.7 mg (2) ⇌ 33.3 mg (1)

(unionised)   (unionised)

Figure 2.1 Simple partition law.

The percentage of drug extracted in the above example is simply given by the mass of drug in the organic phase divided by the total mass of drug, i.e. $66.7/100 = 66.7\%$.

The partition coefficient is an important piece of information as it can be used to predict the absorption, distribution and elimination of drugs within the body. Knowledge of the value of P can be used to predict the onset of action of drugs or the duration of action of drugs, or to tell whether a drug will be active at all. Part of medicinal chemistry, the science of rational drug design, involves structure–activity relationships, where the partition coefficient is used in mathematical equations that try to relate the biological activity of a drug to its physical and chemical characteristics.

In case this sounds too much like an advert for the partition coefficient, in reality the simple relationship above only applies if the solute in question does not ionise at the pH of measurement. If the solute is a weak acid or weak base (and a huge number of drugs are), then ionisation to form a salt will considerably alter the solubility profile of the drug. A fully ionised salt will be much more water soluble than the unionised acid or base, and so the above ratio will vary depending on the pH of measurement.

There are two ways round this problem: either the experimental details are adjusted to ensure that the measured P is the partition coefficient of the unionised molecule (this means that the P value for acids is measured at low pH when the acid is unionised and, similarly, the partition coefficient of a base is measured at high pH to prevent ionisation); or, better, the ratio above is redefined as the *apparent partition coefficient*, to differentiate it from the partition coefficient of the unionised species, which is now termed the *true partition coefficient*.

The apparent partition coefficient (P_{app}) is dependent on the proportion of substance present in solution, which in turn depends upon the pH of the solution, or

$$P_{app} = P \times f_{unionised} \qquad (2.2)$$

where $f_{unionised}$ equals the fraction of the total amount of drug unionised at that pH. It follows that if $f_{unionised} = 1$ then $P_{app} = P_{true}$ and the compound is unionised.

To illustrate the effect of ionisation, consider again the drug in the example above. If the pH of the aqueous phase is adjusted so that the drug becomes 66.7% ionised, only 40 mg of the drug partitions into the organic phase (since the ionised drug will be less soluble in the organic solvent), and the partition coefficient can be recalculated (see Figure 2.2).

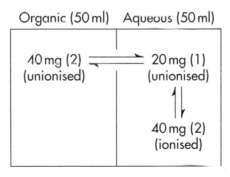

Figure 2.2 The partition of ionised drug.

The mass of drug in the water phase = 100 − 40 = 60 mg.

The mass of ionised drug in the water phase = total mass × fraction ionised, which is 60 × 0.666 = 40 mg.

The mass of unionised drug in the water phase = 60 × 0.333 = 20 mg.

The concentration of drug in the organic phase = 40/50 = 0.8 mg mL^{-1}.

The concentration of unionised drug in the water phase = 20/50 = 0.4 mg mL^{-1}.

The concentration of total drug in the water phase = 60/50 = 1.2 mg mL^{-1}.

The percentage of drug extracted into the organic phase = (40 mg/ 100 mg) × 100 = 40%.

The partition coefficient of the unionised drug (the true partition coefficient) should remain constant and is given by

$$P = \frac{[\text{drug}] \text{ in organic phase}}{[\text{unionised drug}] \text{ in water}}$$

$$P = \frac{0.8 \text{ mg L}^{-1}}{0.4 \text{ mg mL}^{-1}} = 2$$

the same answer as obtained above.

Using the total concentration of drug in the aqueous phase allows the apparent partition coefficient to be calculated:

$$P_{app} = \frac{[\text{drug}] \text{ in organic phase}}{\text{total } [\text{drug}] \text{ in aqueous phase}}$$

$$P_{app} = \frac{0.8 \text{ mg mL}^{-1}}{1.2 \text{ mg mL}^{-1}}$$

$$P_{app} = 0.67$$

The answer for P_{app} can be checked by use of equation (2.2):

$$P_{app} = P \times f_{unionised}$$
$$0.67 = 2 \times 0.33$$

The range of possible values of P found in drug molecules is huge, from small fractions through to values of several thousand. For this reason, it is common to quote the logarithm (to the base 10) of the partition coefficient or log P. This is particularly true in *quantitative structure–activity relationships* (QSAR), where the physicochemical properties of a drug (such as hydrophobicity, steric interactions or electronic effects) are quantified and an equation is derived that can be used to predict the biological activity of other, similar drugs. The technique of QSAR became popular with the advent of powerful computers able to handle the multiple regression analysis necessary to obtain the quite complex equations required. A detailed study of QSAR is beyond the scope of this book, but more advanced textbooks of medicinal chemistry contain many examples of the ability of QSAR equations to predict biological activity.

Experimental measurement of the partition coefficient

There are three convenient ways in which P can be determined in the chemistry laboratory. These are the original *shake flask method*, the use of *thin-layer chromatography* or the use of *reversed-phase, high-performance liquid chromatography*.

Shake flask method

In the shake flask method, the drug whose P is to be determined is traditionally added to a separating funnel containing the two immiscible phases, although it works just as well to use a centrifuge tube (and requires less sample). The two immiscible phases chosen are usually 1-octanol and pH 7.4 buffer. Octanol is used in partition coefficient work because the answers obtained from octanol seem to correlate best with biological data obtained *in vivo*. This may be because the eight carbon atoms are essentially *hydrophobic* (or water-hating) and the one hydroxyl group is *hydrophilic* (water-loving) and together they give the closest balance to that found in human cell membranes. The aqueous buffer at pH 7.4 represents aqueous compartments within the body, e.g. blood plasma.

The two phases are thoroughly mixed to give buffer-saturated octanol in the top phase and octanol-saturated buffer in the bottom. Once the two phases have separated (this can take a while), the drug is added and the whole flask is shaken mechanically for at least an hour. The two phases are allowed to separate (or centrifuged, if you are in a hurry) and the concentration of drug in the aqueous phase is then determined. This may be done by titration if the drug is sufficiently acidic or basic or, more usually, spectrophotometrically. The concentration in the octanol phase is found by subtraction and the value of P is calculated. This method works perfectly well if there is sufficient sample and the drug possesses a chromophore to allow spectroscopic assay of the aqueous phase.

What is important in liquid–liquid extractions of this type is not the volume of the organic phase but rather the number of times the extraction is carried out. Five extractions of 10 mL organic phase will remove more compound than one extraction of 50 mL, even though the total volume of organic solvent used is the same. Similarly, ten extractions of 5 mL will be more efficient still, and so on. This effect (which is general to all extractions) is obvious when thought about. Each time one phase is removed and replaced by fresh solvent, the equilibrium for the partitioning process must re-establish according to the partition coefficient ratio and drug must leave the aqueous phase to enter the organic phase and restore the equilibrium ratio.

An equation can be derived to calculate the increase in efficiency of multiple extractions versus one single extraction:

$$W_n = W \left(\frac{A}{PS + A} \right)^n \tag{2.3}$$

where W_n is the mass of drug remaining in the aqueous phase after n extractions, W is the initial mass of drug in the aqueous phase, A is the volume of the aqueous phase, S is the volume of solvent (or organic) phase, P is the partition coefficient and n is the number of extractions.

Equation (2.3) is derived as follows:

$$P = \frac{[\text{organic}]}{[\text{aqueous}]}$$

or, using the terms defined above,

$$P = \frac{(W - W_1)/S}{(W_1/A)}$$

Therefore,

$$P = \frac{(W - W_1)}{W_1} \times \frac{A}{S}$$

or

$$\frac{PS}{A} = \frac{(W - W_1)}{W_1} = \frac{W}{W_1} - 1$$

Hence,

$$\frac{W}{W_1} = \frac{PS}{A} + 1 = \frac{PS}{A} + \frac{A}{A}$$

Therefore, the fraction of drug remaining in the aqueous phase is

$$\frac{W_1}{W} = \frac{A}{(PS + A)} \tag{2.4}$$

This expression is valid for one extraction; it follows that if the extraction is repeated n times, the overall expression is simply given by equation (2.4) repeated n times, which, with subscript 1 replaced by n, is equation (2.3).

Thin-layer chromatography (TLC)

In this technique, the R_f value of the drug is related mathematically to the partition coefficient. A thin-layer plate, or a paper sheet, is pre-coated with organic phase (usually paraffin or octanol) and allowed to dry. Sample is applied to the origin and the plate is allowed to develop. The mobile phase used is either water or a mixture of water and a miscible organic solvent (such as acetone) to improve the solubility of the drug.

Once the plate has developed, the spots are visualised (using an ultraviolet lamp if the drug possesses a chromophore, or iodine vapour if it does not) and the R_f for each spot is determined. The R_f is the distance moved by the spot divided by the distance moved by the solvent front, and is expressed as a decimal. The R_f can be related to the partition coefficient by equations of the type

$$P = \frac{k}{(1/R_f) - 1} \qquad (2.5)$$

where k is a constant for the given system, which is determined by running a number of standard compounds of known P in the system and calculating k.

The TLC method of determining P works best for compounds of similar structure and physical properties. The advantages of using this technique to determine P are that many compounds can be run simultaneously on one plate, and very little sample is required. On the other hand, finding suitable standards can be difficult, and aqueous mobile phases can take many hours to run up a large TLC plate.

High-performance liquid chromatography (HPLC)

This method of analysis relies on the same chemical principles as the determination by TLC, except that the efficiency (and the cost) of the technique has increased greatly. Instead of the R_f value, the retention time of the drug is measured and related to P by equations similar to equation (2.5) for TLC. The retention time, as its name suggests, is the time taken for the sample to elute from the HPLC column. The major drawback with using this technique to determine P is detecting the drug if it does not possess a chromophore, when a UV detector cannot be used. In cases like this, use must be made of an HPLC system connected to a refractive index (RI) detector or an electrochemical detector (ECD). A RI detector relies on changes in the refractive index of the mobile phase as a solute elutes to detect a signal, while an ECD functions like a little electrode to oxidise or reduce the analyte as it elutes. In either case, before the determination of P is carried out, you should seriously consider measuring P for another drug! My PhD supervisor had a saying: 'Never make a compound you cannot name'; to that can be added the advice 'Never make a compound that cannot be detected by a UV detector.' Many entertaining hours can be spent optimising HPLC systems with RI or ECD, but if you want to finish before your children grow up, these methods of detection are best avoided.

There are some advantages to the HPLC method of determining P, namely that HPLC does not require much sample and that the sample does not have to be 100% pure. Also, once the complete system has been obtained, the cost of the determination is limited to the purchase of HPLC-grade solvents and electricity.

Drug absorption and distribution

The most popular method of administering drugs and medicines, at least in the UK, is the oral route. Tablets, capsules or oral liquids are swallowed and, once in the stomach, the tablet or capsule disintegrates to release the active drug molecule. Interestingly, a drug is not considered to be *in* the body until it has been absorbed across the gut wall and into the bloodstream. The gut can be thought of as a hollow tube running through the body, open at both ends (hopefully not at the same time) and, as such, the gut contents are considered *outside* the body. Passage into the body must be achieved by absorption across a biological membrane; for the oral route of drug administration, this is the cell membrane of cells lining the wall of the stomach and the intestine. Once the drug has passed through the gut membrane into the bloodstream, it then has to travel to its site of action and diffuse out of the bloodstream to the receptor on some, perhaps distant, cell membrane.

In the case of drugs acting on the brain or spinal cord (the central nervous system, or CNS) the drug must partition across the *blood–brain barrier* to gain access to the CNS. The blood–brain barrier is, in reality, the cell membranes of glial cells (or *astrocytes*) lining the blood vessels within the brain. These cells fuse together very closely to form a very tight, high-resistance 'lipid barrier' that restricts the passage of many drug molecules, especially if the drug molecules are polar. It has been estimated that the blood–brain barrier prevents the brain uptake of >98% of all potential neurotherapeutics. This barrier is designed to protect the delicate structures of the brain from damage by harmful compounds that may gain access to the bloodstream, but it can be a problem for drug administration. Some infectious diseases, such as malaria, can spread to the brain and, once established, can be very difficult to treat, since drugs used to eradicate the infection in other parts of the body cannot cross the blood–brain barrier to get at the infection in the CNS. A similarly depressing picture exists with brain tumours. Conventional anticancer chemotherapy often cannot penetrate the barrier to attack the tumour. All of the small polar molecules (e.g. amino acids, sugars) required by the brain have their own transport proteins located at the blood–brain barrier that act to transfer the essential compound through the barrier in a process called carrier-mediated transport.

Biological membranes vary in structure and function throughout the body, but there are some common structural features and properties (see Figure 2.3). A cell membrane is composed of a bilayer of fatty molecules known as phospholipids. These compounds are amphoteric in nature, possessing a non-polar region of hydrocarbon chains that are buried inside the cell membrane, and a polar region comprising negatively charged phosphoric acid head groups. These ionised groups are exposed to the aqueous surroundings of the extracellular and intracellular fluids of the cell. The cell membrane has to be fatty and non-polar in nature to allow it to successfully separate the aqueous compartments of the body. Buried within this lipid bilayer are large globular protein molecules. These macromolecules function as ion channels (e.g. the Na^+ channel of nerve membranes), transmembrane receptors (like the β receptor) or transport proteins (as in the electron transport chain of mitochondria). Human cell membranes also contain high concentrations of the steroid cholesterol, particularly in nerve tissue. Chemically, cholesterol is a cyclopentanoperhydrophenanthrene derivative, but it is much simpler to call this important group of compounds with this tetracyclic nucleus 'steroids.' The structure of cholesterol and a general structure of membrane phospholipids are shown in Figure 2.4.

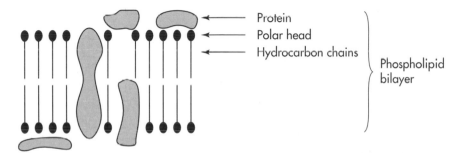

Figure 2.3 A fluid mosaic model of a cell membrane.

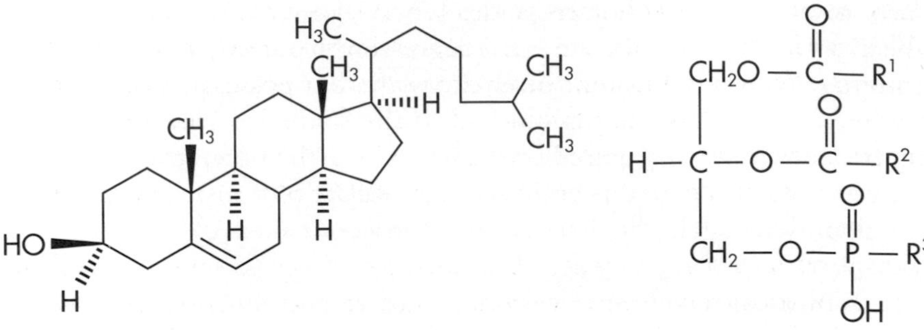

Figure 2.4　The structures of cholesterol and phospholipids. R^1 and R^2 = palmityl, stearyl or oleyl. R^3 = ethanolamine, choline, serine, inositol or glycerol.

Cholesterol gets a bad press nowadays. Tabloid newspapers and television programmes seem to have latched onto cholesterol as the villain of a healthy lifestyle. It is true that high levels of cholesterol in the diet, coupled with high salt intake and lack of exercise, are blamed for causing coronary heart disease and strokes. In cell membranes, however, cholesterol increases membrane rigidity and is essential for maintaining the integrity of the membrane – without cholesterol your cells would leak. Other important steroids include the male sex hormone, testosterone, and the female sex hormones oestrogen and progestogen in addition to drugs such as digoxin and beclometasone.

For a small drug molecule to travel across membranes of this type, one of two things must happen: either the drug must cross the membrane by passive diffusion down a concentration gradient or the drug has to be transported across the membrane, against the concentration gradient, with the expenditure of energy (active transport).

Passive diffusion

Passive diffusion is probably the most important mechanism by which small drug molecules gain access to the body. The drug molecule must be in solution and it partitions into the lipophilic cell membrane, diffuses across the cell and then partitions out of cell and into the aqueous compartment on the other side. Drugs that are very lipid soluble, (such as the antifungal agent griseofulvin) are so water insoluble that they partition into the cell membrane but then stick in the lipid membrane and do not partition out of the membrane and into the aqueous compartments inside the cell. Similarly, drugs that are very water soluble will not partition well into a non-polar lipid membrane and will tend to stay in the aqueous contents of the gut. Clearly, for a drug to be successfully absorbed from the gut it must possess an intermediate level of water solubility and lipid solubility: a sort of 'Goldilocks effect', where the drug is not too hydrophobic, not too hydrophilic, but possesses just the right degree of solubility to partition through biological membranes. In general, drugs that are strongly acidic ($pK_a < 2$) or basic ($pK_a > 10$) will not cross membranes very well since they will be >99.99% ionised at the pH of the gut.

Transfer across membranes occurs down a concentration gradient (i.e. from regions of high drug concentration to regions where the concentration is lower). The process of diffusion can be described by Fick's law, which states

$$\frac{dm}{dt} = \frac{PDA(C_2 - C_1)}{d}$$

where dm/dt is the rate of appearance of drug within the cell (or rate of transfer), P is the partition coefficient of the drug, D is a diffusion coefficient for the membrane, A is the surface area of membrane available for absorption, C_2 and C_1 are the concentrations of drug on the external and internal surfaces, respectively, and d is the thickness of the cell membrane.

Passive diffusion can only occur with small molecules (e.g. drugs with relative molecular masses of approximately 1000 or less). This excludes large macromolecules such as proteins, which are polyelectrolytes and do not partition well across lipid membranes. This can be important for drugs that are extensively bound to proteins in the bloodstream. These drugs are effectively trapped in the blood plasma and cannot easily gain access into and through cells. The effect is most noticeable for drugs that do not distribute widely around the body and are highly bound to plasma proteins (>90% of the given dose). Examples of these include the anticoagulant warfarin, the antibacterial sulfonamides and oral hypoglycaemic drugs such as tolbutamide.

The potential for serious drug interactions occurs with drugs bound to plasma proteins. The binding sites on the protein molecule are relatively non-specific, and a bound drug can easily be displaced by another drug with affinity for the protein. The well-documented interaction between the anticoagulant warfarin and non-steroidal anti-inflammatory drugs (NSAIDs) such as aspirin, indometacin and phenylbutazone arises in this way. When warfarin is administered, >90% of the dose can circulate in the blood bound to plasma proteins; this means that the patient is effectively stabilised on the remaining 10% of the dose of drug. If aspirin is co-administered with warfarin, the aspirin can displace warfarin from binding sites on the protein and increase the 'effective' concentration of warfarin in the body, leading to decreases in clotting time and haemorrhage. This serious effect is potentiated by inhibition of the metabolism of warfarin by NSAIDs.

The pH partition hypothesis

Biological membranes are, essentially, non-polar or hydrophobic, due to the long hydrocarbon chains of the phospholipid molecules. For a drug to cross a membrane of this type, the drug must pass from the aqueous solution of the extracellular fluid, through the lipid membrane to the aqueous solution of the intracellular fluid (see Figure 2.5), i.e. the drug must be sufficiently soluble in both the aqueous and the lipid phases to succeed.

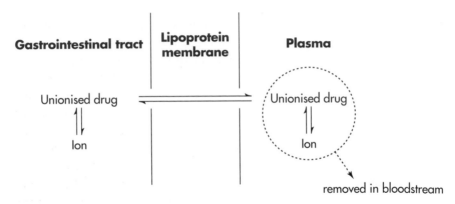

Figure 2.5 A partition diagram of a cell membrane.

For any given drug (or, for that matter, for any biological membrane) there must exist an optimal value of partition coefficient for transport of drug across the membrane. This value is called P_0.

The situation becomes (even) more complicated if the drug ionises at the pH of the body compartment. For weak acids and weak bases, the aqueous and lipid solubility of the compound will depend on the extent to which the drug is ionised, which in turn will depend on the pK_a of the acidic and basic groups involved and the pH of the surroundings.

For weak acids that ionise as

$$HA \rightleftharpoons H^+ + A^-$$

the unionised species, HA, will be much more lipid soluble, and will therefore cross biological membranes much more rapidly than will the anion A⁻. This suggests that weak acids will be absorbed more efficiently across a membrane when the pH of the surrounding solution is low and the weak acid will be predominantly unionised. Such a situation is found in the gastric juice of the stomach, which, due to the high concentration of hydrochloric acid present, is at a pH of 1–2 (this is why gastric ulcers are so painful: the hole in the gut lining allows the acid to burn the underlying muscle layer). This theory is called the *pH partition hypothesis*, and predicts that weakly acidic drugs such as aspirin, barbiturates, phenytoin, etc. will be absorbed preferentially from the stomach rather than from the more alkaline small intestine. In a region of high pH, the acidic drug will ionise to give A⁻, which, since it is charged, will not diffuse well through a hydrophobic lipid membrane.

For weak bases that ionise as

$$B + H_2O \rightleftharpoons BH^+ + OH^-$$

the more lipid-soluble species is the unionised free base, B, which will be present to the greatest extent in solutions of high pH, such as are found in the small intestine (pH range 6–8). The pH partition hypothesis predicts that basic drugs (such as morphine, codeine, antihistamines, etc.) will be absorbed into the body better from the small intestine than from the acidic stomach, where the base will be present mainly as the ionised conjugate acid. This is important for the patient, since, if a drug can only be absorbed from the small intestine, there will inevitably be a delay in onset of action if the drug is taken orally. The drug has to be swallowed and pass through the stomach (where if it is basic it will exist predominantly in the ionised form) before the stomach empties and the drug enters the small intestine and begins the process of absorption. If, for example, a patient takes a basic drug such as an antihistamine for travel sickness, they should be advised to swallow their medication at least an hour before they set off on their journey to allow time for the drug to reach the site of absorption and partition into the bloodstream.

An estimate of the extent to which a weak acid or base will be ionised at any given pH can be made using the approximate 'rule of thumb' introduced in Chapter 1 if the pK_a of the acid or base is known.

Limitations of the pH partition hypothesis

The pH partition hypothesis is very useful as a model to explain the extent of drug absorption in the body, but it must be borne in mind that the model has some limitations. As usual, the real-life situation is more complex than this simple model allows for. Although the theory predicts that weak acids will preferentially be absorbed from the stomach, and weak bases from the small intestine, in reality the vast majority of drugs are absorbed from the small intestine irrespective of their degree of ionisation. This is because the small intestine is designed as the organ where absorption of food (and drugs) takes place. The small intestine has three sections, the *duodenum*, a short curved section attached to the back wall of the abdomen, and the *jejunum* and *ileum*, two larger coiled segments that can move about within the abdominal cavity. The existenceof these three sections means that the small intestine is long (about 6.5 metres in an adult) and has much higher surface area (estimated as 100 m²) than the stomach. The large intestine, which frames the coils of the small intestine, follows on from the small intestine and is itself about 1.5 metres long. This means the total length of the gut is over 8 metres, or approximately six times an individual's height. The high surface area of the small intestine is achieved due to its convoluted folded structure (see Figure 2.6), which is increased further by the presence of *microvilli*, small tube-like structures, like tiny hairs, which extend into the gut lumen. The small intestine is also supplied with a rich blood supply, which means that food or drug molecules, once they cross the gut membrane, are carried away in the bloodstream initially to the liver, and from there are distributed around the body.

What all this means in practice is that drugs are absorbed quite effectively from the small intestine even if they exist in a predominantly ionised form. The absorption process obeys the *law of mass action*, which was introduced in Chapter 1. This law is fundamentally an equilibrium process, and, as with any equilibrium, rapid removal of the 'products' or compounds on the right-hand side of the equilibrium arrow will shift the equilibrium in that direction. This is exactly what happens in drug absorption across the gut membrane: a small amount of unionised drug is absorbed by passive diffusion and whisked away by the rich blood supply of the gut. This allows the equilibrium to re-establish, and more drug to be absorbed. In this way, acidic or basic drugs, which may be >99% ionised at the pH of the gut, may be absorbed quite effectively into the body.

Some ionised drug molecules can traverse the lipophilic gut membrane by combining with an ion of opposite charge (a *counter ion*) to form an ion pair. The ion pair, although composed of two ionic species, behaves as a neutral molecule with a high partition coefficient and can

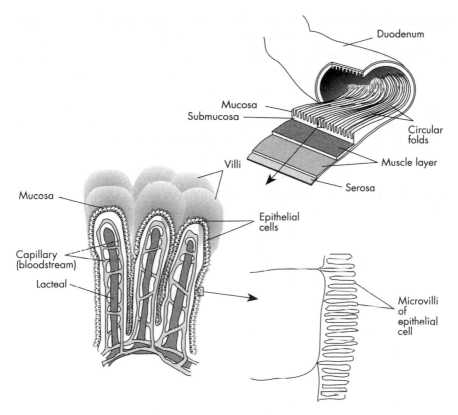

Figure 2.6 A diagram of the small intestine, showing the convoluted surface made up of villi, which are lined with microvilli.

cross biomembranes effectively. Quaternary ammonium compounds may be absorbed in this way:

$$N^+R_4 + A^- \rightleftharpoons [N^+R_4A^-] \qquad \text{easily absorbed ion pair}$$

Active transport mechanisms

Occasionally, a chemical is so essential to the functioning of the body that special mechanisms are established to allow the essential molecules or ions to cross cell membranes. Glucose and ions such as sodium and chloride must cross membranes efficiently, but they are too polar to diffuse across a phospholipid bilayer passively. Their transport is 'facilitated' by proteins that span the membrane and allow these chemicals to enter cells. If the transport occurs down a concentration gradient, the process is described as *facilitated diffusion* and does not usually require expenditure of energy in the form of hydrolysis of ATP (adenosine triphosphate). The protein merely aids the uptake process by allowing an alternative route of access (this mechanism includes gated hydrophilic pores, such as ion channels, which are discussed below). In the alternative process where the transport occurs against an existing concentration gradient, the process is defined as *active transport* and does require metabolic energy to be expended in the form of hydrolysis of ATP to ADP (adenosine diphosphate). A good example of this type of active transport occurs with amino acids. As discussed in Chapter 1, amino acids are the monomers from which proteins are made and exist predominantly as the zwitterion at neutral pH. This 'internal salt' is far too hydrophilic to partition through a lipophilic lipid membrane by passive diffusion, so energy generated from the oxidation of food must be used in order to ensure that these essential molecules are absorbed from the diet. The active transport mechanism usually involves a 'carrier' molecule, which 'recognises' the desired compound and forms a complex with it at the cell surface. These carrier molecules are proteins in nature and are specific for the molecule in question. The protein complex diffuses across the cell membrane and, once on the other side, dissociates to release the compound. The carrier protein is then free to return to the outside of the cell membrane to pick up another molecule to transport. A drug that is similar in structure to an essential natural compound can, in some cases, fool the transport mechanism and be absorbed actively into the body. The anticancer drug *melphalan* was synthesised in order to make use of the existing active transport pathway for the amino acid phenylalanine (see Figure 2.7). The phenyl-

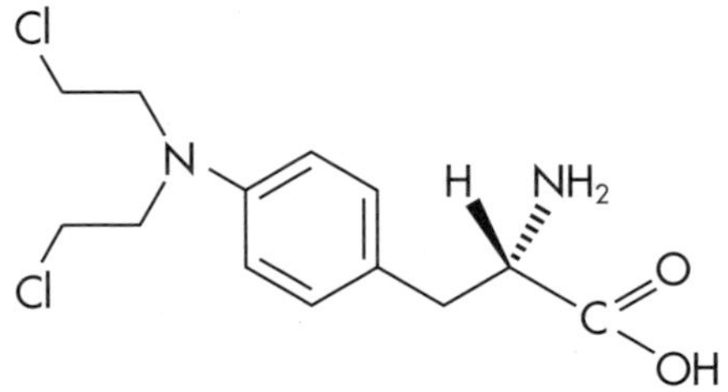

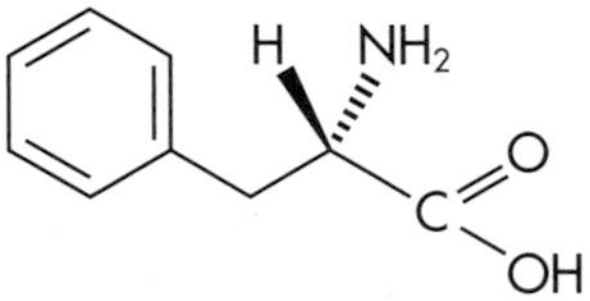

Figure 2.7 The structures of melphalan and phenylalanine.

alanine part of the molecule takes no part in the anticancer action, it is merely there to improve the molecule's chances of being absorbed across biomembranes. Interestingly, only the natural L-phenylalanine analogue is absorbed actively, the opposite D form is only absorbed slowly by passive diffusion. This fact neatly illustrates that active transport, like most of the body's biochemical mechanisms, is chiral in nature, and can easily discriminate between enantiomers.

The action of local anaesthetics

The physicochemical properties of drugs that underlie their absorption within the body can be complex, and the pH partition hypothesis is not sufficiently comprehensive to explain all the processes that occur *in vivo*; it is, however, a good place to start. Perhaps surprisingly for such a simple theory, the pH partition hypothesis can explain quite complicated pharmacological observations. The processes that occur when a patient swallows a tablet are so complicated that the most powerful computers known to science cannot adequately model the process. It is astonishing, therefore, that a few physicochemical constants (pK_a and partition coefficient, for example) can provide useful information and, when used properly, predict the possibility and extent of drug absorption.

An example of drug action that can be adequately explained by the pH partition hypothesis, is the mechanism(s) of action of local anaesthetic drugs. Local anaesthetics are drugs that are used to induce a state of temporary analgesia, or freedom from pain. They achieve this by blocking the conduction of impulses along nerve fibres responsible for the transmission of painful stimuli from a site of an injury to the brain and CNS.

Local anaesthetics are basic drugs, all derived originally from cocaine (see Figure 2.8), an alkaloid obtained from the leaves of the shrub *Erythroxylum coca*, which grows wild in the Andes region of South America. Cocaine is a very effective local anaesthetic, but due to a profound stimulant action on the CNS, it has been replaced in most routine procedures with synthetic, non-addictive, analogues such as lidocaine (lignocaine), prilocaine, procaine, etc. These drugs are aliphatic amines, with pK_a values for their conjugate acids of approximately 8–9. Applying the 'rule of thumb' shows that local anaesthetics will exist approximately 99% ionised at blood pH (7.4).

The site of action of most local anaesthetics is a Na^+ ion channel found in the cell membrane of nerve cells (or *neurons*). This Na^+ channel, as its name suggests, allows Na^+ ions to travel through the cell

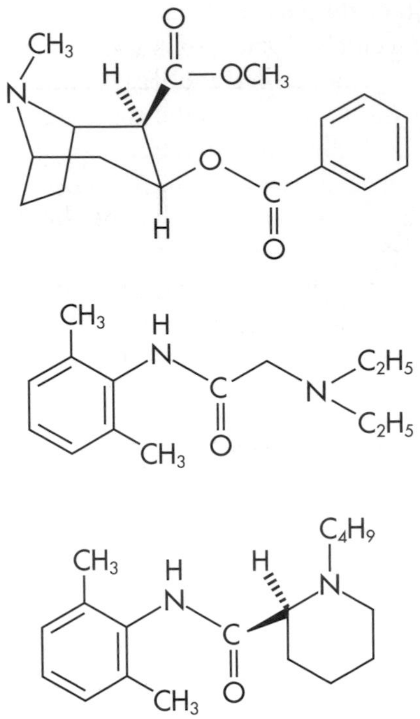

Cocaine

lidocaine (lignocaine)

Bupivacaine

Figure 2.8 The structures of cocaine, lidocaine (lignocaine) and bupivacaine.

membrane to depolarise the resting membrane potential and allow the nerve cell to fire. Local anaesthetics block nerve conduction by attaching to the protein of the Na^+ channel and disrupting the flow of Na^+ ions. Recent research using radiolabelled local anaesthetics has shown that the local anaesthetic attaches to a structure at the *intracellular* opening of the Na^+ channel, and that the form of the drug active at the receptor is the positively charged *conjugate acid*, which prompts the question 'How does an ionised drug get to the internal opening of the ion channel?' The apparently obvious answer is that the cationic form of the local anaesthetic gains entry to the nerve cell by the same route as the Na^+ ions, i.e. down the open sodium channel. Although this may explain part of local anaesthetic action, it cannot be the full story, since most local anaesthetics are too large to pass through the channel. The answer lies within the properties of equilibria and can be predicted from the pH partition hypothesis (see Figure 2.9).

The important thing to remember in this situation is that although 99 out of every 100 local anaesthetic molecules are ionised, there exists

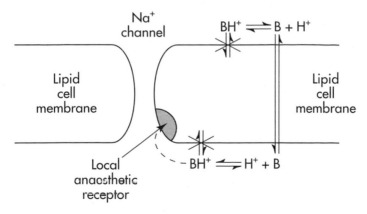

Figure 2.9   A diagram of local anaesthetic equilibrium.

an equilibrium between the cation and the unionised free base. This unionised free base (B) can diffuse easily through the cell membrane, where it will become instantly ionised due to the H^+ ions present within the cell. Once ionised to the cation (BH^+), the local anaesthetic cannot easily diffuse back outside the cell, but it can approach the receptor situated at the internal opening of the sodium channel. Once the 1% of free base has diffused into the cell, *the equilibrium must re-establish to give a further 1% free base*. This unionised free base can diffuse into the cell easily, the equilibrium re-establishes, and so on. These so called 'sink conditions' mean that a substantial portion of a drug dose can reach the site of action even though, at first glance, there appears to be insufficient unionised drug to partition across the membrane. This system is an example of a *dynamic equilibrium* and should be studied carefully. Dynamic equilibria occur in many sites in the body and are responsible for a significant amount of drug absorption.

Excretion and reabsorption of drugs

Previously in this chapter, the pH partition hypothesis was applied to the absorption of drugs across biological membranes following administration by the oral route. The same types of physicochemical processes occur when drugs are reabsorbed into the bloodstream following excretion by the kidneys.

The two kidneys are situated at the back of the abdomen on either side of the vertebral column. They carry out many functions in the body, the most important of which is the production of urine and the excretion from the body of low molecular weight (relative molecular mass less than 68 000) water-soluble compounds, including many drugs. Each kidney contains approximately one million urine-producing structures called nephrons. The nephron in turn consists of a bundle of blood capillaries termed a *glomerulus*, which functions as a very efficient filter to remove waste products and impurities from the blood, and a long tube-like structure called a *tubule* (see Figure 2.10).

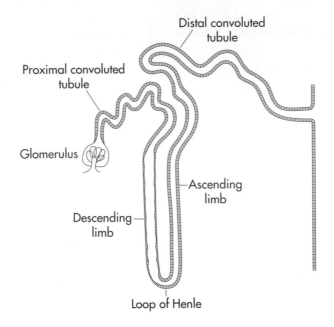

Figure 2.10 A diagram of a nephron.

The kidneys receive a large blood flow (approximately a quarter of the total cardiac output of 5 litres per minute) and from this volume of blood approximately 170 litres of filtrate are produced every day. Clearly, the body would quickly become dehydrated if this volume of fluid were lost to the sewage system, so most of it is reabsorbed from the kidney tubule and returned to the bloodstream. Small molecules that are dissolved in the glomerular filtrate are also reabsorbed back into the bloodstream, either by passive diffusion (which obeys Fick's law) or by the utilisation of energy in an active transport process similar to the mechanisms for gut absorption discussed previously. It should be realised that reabsorption from the glomerular filtrate and return to the bloodstream are involved in the duration of action of many drugs, and a drug molecule may be filtered and reabsorbed many times before it is finally excreted from the body.

In cases of drug overdose it is desirable to eliminate the toxic drug from the body as quickly as possible and techniques have been evolved to minimise the process of reabsorption of drug from the kidney tubule and so expedite excretion. If a drug is to be reabsorbed by passive diffusion through the tubule cell membrane, then it must exist predominately in the *unionised* form. This is entirely in keeping with the process of absorption into the body following oral administration discussed above. If the pH of the urine is adjusted to increase the proportion of the drug that is ionised, then reabsorption will be decreased (since the unionised species crosses the membrane more easily by passive diffusion).

If the drug taken in overdose is a weak acid (e.g. a barbiturate, phenytoin, most NSAIDs) then excretion should be favoured, and reabsorption minimised, by addition of an agent that will raise the pH of the urine. This technique is called *forced alkaline diuresis* and should result in more rapid clearance of an acidic drug. An example of an agent used to raise the pH of urine is sodium bicarbonate, $Na^+HCO_3^-$ (the salt of a strong base and a weak acid, which will be basic by partial hydrolysis), usually administered as an 8.4% w/v infusion.

If the drug taken in overdose is a base, for example, a benzodiazepine tranquilliser or an antihistamine, excretion should be favoured by acidification of the urine. Agents that may be used to achieve this include ammonium chloride, $NH_4^+Cl^-$ (an acidic salt by partial hydrolysis) and ascorbic acid (vitamin C). If the pH of the urine is artificially lowered, the technique is called *forced acid diuresis*.

Food and drink

Solubility and partition effects do not only occur with drug molecules. In everyday life, the effects of water solubility, or lack of it, can be observed. This can be neatly illustrated using two consumables familiar to generations of students, namely alcohol and curry!

In France, it is the custom before a meal to partake of an aperitif, usually an aniseed-flavoured spirit called *pastis*. Pastis (e.g. 'Ricard', 'Pernod') when it comes out of the bottle is a clear, light brown coloured solution of volatile oils from the seeds of the anise plant (*Pimpinella anisum*), which impart the characteristic aniseed flavour to the drink, dissolved in approximately 40% v/v ethanol. When a pastis is drunk, it is mixed with water and ice, whereupon the liquid becomes cloudy. This happens because the anise oils are hydrophobic, non-polar liquids and not very water-soluble. They are only held in solution by the high alcohol content of the drink. When the alcohol is diluted with water, the oils come out of solution and form an emulsion of oil droplets in the aqueous phase. This is what gives the drink its cloudy appearance. Oral solutions of anise oils have been used pharmaceutically for their carminative action and as an aid to digestion for many years, although it seems to this author preferable to consume anise oils in the form of a pastis, rather than in the form of a bottle of medicine.

Spicy foods such as curries and chillies and flavourings such as tabasco and paprika derive their hot pungent taste from the compound *capsaicin* (Figure 2.11). Capsaicin is found in the fruits of various species of *Capsicum* and is a powerful irritant causing intense pain if administered in a pure form. As can be seen from Figure 2.11, capsaicin is a non-polar compound possessing few polar groups to hydrogen bond to water. This means that capsaicin is virtually insoluble in water. This is important information for people who eat spicy food. If a curry or chilli is too hot there is little point in trying to counteract the burning in your mouth by consuming water (or beer!) as capsaicin is not soluble in aqueous solution. A far better strategy to put out the fire is to consume a non-aqueous liquid such as milk (an oil in water emulsion) in which the capsaicin can dissolve. Alternatively, eating a fatty food such as bread with butter can help the capsaicin partition into the fat on the bread rather than the lipid of your epithelium. Incidentally, the temperature of the mouth does not increase while eating a hot, spicy meal, even though you may feel warm as a result. Capsaicin is a chemical irritant and does not raise the temperature of the mouth at all.

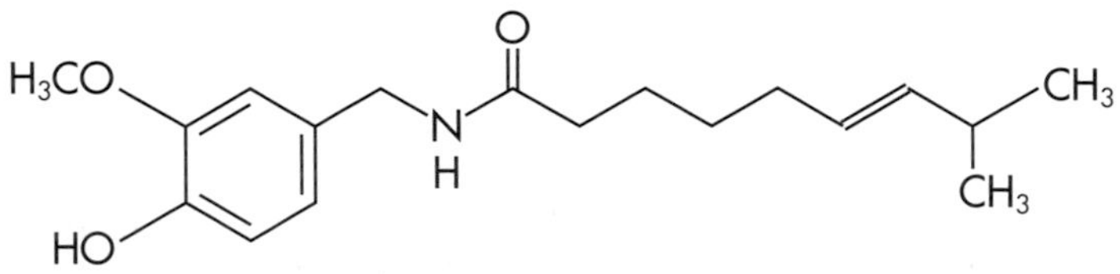

Figure 2.11 The structure of capsaicin.

The irritant properties of capsaicin are employed in pharmacological research, where it is used to stimulate sensory nerves and as an experimental treatment for chronic pain. Patients suffering intense chronic pain that cannot be treated by analgesics may gain some relief by the use of capsaicin, which destroys the sensory nerves carrying the painful stimulus. Capsaicin is also used for more sinister purposes. A solution of capsaicin (pepper spray) is used by police forces around the world as a non-lethal weapon to temporarily blind and incapacitate criminals resisting arrest.

Tutorial examples

1 *A basic drug, pK$_a$ = 9.4, P = 65, was administered to a patient and 5 mL of blood plasma was removed for analysis. This 5 mL of sample was extracted with 10 mL of octanol and the concentration of drug in the octanol was found to be 34 ng mL^{-1}. Calculate the following:*
(a)   The apparent partition coefficient at pH 7.4
(b)   The concentration of drug in plasma before extraction
(c)   The percentage of drug extracted in a single extraction

1   The first step is to calculate the fraction of the drug unionised at pH 7.4. The equation for the percentage ionised for a base is

$$\% \text{ Ionised} = \frac{100}{1 + \text{antilog} (\text{pH} - pK_a)}$$

$$\% \text{ Ionised} = \frac{100}{1 + \text{antilog} (7.4 - 9.4)}$$

$$\% \text{ Ionised} = 99\%$$

Therefore, the percentage unionised = 1% and the fraction unionised = 1/100 = 0.01.

$$P_{\text{app}} = P \times \text{fraction unionised}$$
$$P_{\text{app}} = 65 \times 0.01$$
$$P_{\text{app}} = 0.65$$

(b)   Before we can calculate the concentration of drug in the plasma *before* the extraction, we have to consider the concentration present *after* the extraction and remember that all of the drug in the octanol and the plasma started off in the plasma. Thus,

$$P_{\text{app}} = \frac{\text{concentration in octanol after extraction}}{\text{concentration in plasma after extraction}}$$

$$P_{\text{app}} = \frac{34 \text{ ng mL}^{-1}}{\text{plasma concentration}}$$

$$0.65 = \frac{34 \text{ ng mL}^{-1}}{\text{plasma concentration}}$$

Concentration in plasma after extraction = 52.3 ng mL^{-1}

To calculate the concentration of drug in the plasma *before* the extraction, we have to convert the concentrations into amounts (i.e. mass) of drug.

The amount of drug in octanol *after* extraction is volume × concentration = 10 × 34 = 340 ng.

The amount of drug in plasma *after* extraction is volume × concentration = 5 × 52.3 = 261.5 ng.

The total amount of drug in the initial plasma sample = 340 + 261.5 = 601.5 ng.

Therefore the *initial* concentration of drug in plasma is given by

$$\frac{\text{Amount}}{\text{Volume}} = \frac{601.5}{5} = 120.3 \text{ ng mL}^{-1}$$

(c) The percentage extracted in a single extraction is easily calculated from the following.

The amount extracted into octanol = 340 ng.

The total amount of drug in plasma = 601.5 ng.

Therefore,

$$\% \text{ Extracted} = \left(\frac{340}{601.5}\right) \times 100 = 56.5\%$$

Q 2 *5.0 mL of a plasma sample (pH 7.4) containing an acidic drug (pK$_a$ = 6.5) was extracted with 10.0 mL of ether. The concentration of drug in both layers was determined and the results obtained were:*

The total concentration (unionised + ionised) in plasma = 16 μg mL^{-1}
The concentration in ether = 7 μg mL^{-1}

From these data determine the following:
(a) The distribution of the drug between the two phases at equilibrium
(b) The apparent partition coefficient, P$_{app}$
(c) The partition coefficient, P
(d) The percentage extracted
(e) How the efficiency of the extraction might be improved by modification of the pH
(f) The percentage extracted under the modified conditions

2(a) From the pK_a value and the pH it can be seen that the acidic drug will be ionised at plasma pH.

$$\% \text{ Ionised for an acid} = \frac{100}{1 + \text{antilog}\,(pK_a - pH)}$$

$$= \frac{100}{1 + \text{antilog}\,(6.5 - 7.4)}$$

$$= 88.8\%$$

Thus, the fraction ionised $(f_i) = 0.888$.
Therefore, the fraction unionised $(f_u) = 1 - 0.888 = 0.112$.

Mass of drug in ether $= 7\ \mu g\ mL^{-1} \times 10\ mL = 70\ \mu g$

Mass of drug in the plasma $= 16\ \mu g\ mL^{-1} \times 5\ mL = 80\ \mu g$

Amount of drug ionised $= 0.888 \times 80\ \mu g = 71\ \mu g$

Amount of drug unionised $= 0.112 \times 80\ \mu g = 9\ \mu g$

Amount of drug in the total system $= 70\ \mu g + 80\ \mu g$
$= 150\ \mu g$

(b) P_{app} can be calculated from the concentration data since the drug is ionised in the plasma.

$$P_{app} = \frac{[\text{drug}]\ \text{in ether}}{\text{total}\ [\text{drug}]\ \text{in plasma}}$$

$$= \frac{7\ \mu g\ mL^{-1}}{16\ \mu g\ mL^{-1}}$$

$$= 0.44$$

(c) The partition coefficient, P, is given by

$$P = \frac{P_{app}}{\text{fraction unionised}}$$

$$= 0.44 / 0.112$$

$$= 3.93$$

It should be noted that P is greater than P_{app} since the drug will be ionised at the pH of measurement of P_{app} and hence will be less soluble in the ether phase.

(d)   The percentage of drug extracted is given by

$$\frac{\text{Mass of drug in ether}}{\text{Total mass of drug in system}}$$

$$= \frac{70\ \mu g}{150\ \mu g} \times 100$$

$$= 47\%$$

(e)   Since the drug is an acid, lowering of the pH of the plasma sample (e.g. by the addition of a small volume of strong acid) will suppress ionisation of the drug and allow more drug to partition into the ether phase.

(f)   If the plasma sample is acidified so that $P_{app} = P = 3.93$, the mass of drug extracted when it is essentially unionised can be calculated. The mass of drug remaining in the plasma after extraction under the new conditions is $x\ \mu g$. Therefore, the mass extracted into the ether $= (150 - x)\ \mu g$.

$$\text{Concentration of drug in plasma} = \frac{x}{5}\ \mu g\ mL^{-1}$$

$$\text{Concentration of drug in ether} = \frac{(150 - x)}{10}\ \mu g\ mL^{-1}$$

$$P = \frac{[\text{drug}]\ \text{in ether}}{[\text{drug}]\ \text{in plasma}}$$

$$= \frac{(150 - x)/10}{x/5}$$

$$= 3.93$$

When this unpleasant looking piece of algebra is solved for x, we obtain

$$\text{Mass of drug remaining in plasma} = 17\ \mu g$$
$$\text{Mass of drug extracted into the ether} = (150 - 17)\ \mu g$$
$$= 133\ \mu g$$
$$\%\ \text{Extracted under new conditions} = (133/150) \times 100$$
$$= 89\%$$

which shows, as expected, that acidification of the plasma sample increases the percentage extracted from 47% to 89%.

Problems

Q2.1 Explain the difference between the true partition coefficient and the apparent partition coefficient.

Outline how the true partition coefficient of a sparingly water-soluble drug such as sulfamethoxazole might conveniently be measured (see Figure 2.12).

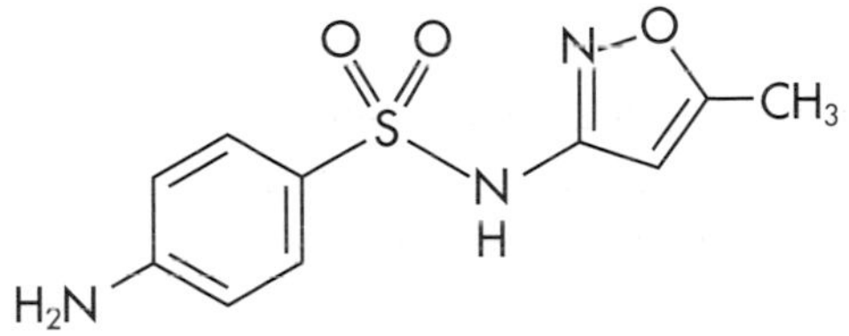

Figure 2.12 The structure of sulfamethoxazole, pK_a = 5.6, P (ether : water) = 125.

A 4 mL aliquot of plasma (pH 7.4) was taken from a patient receiving treatment with sulfamethoxazole and extracted with 2 × 5 mL aliquots of ether. The ether extracts were combined, evaporated to dryness and reconstituted in 2 mL of chloroform. The concentration of sulfamethoxazole in the chloroform was found to be 15.8 μg mL^{-1}. Calculate the original concentration of drug in the plasma sample.

What percentage of the drug was extracted in the procedure outlined above and how might the procedure be changed to increase this value?

Q2.2 The structure of the β-blocker atenolol (pK_a 9.6, P (ether : water) 275) is shown in Figure 2.13.

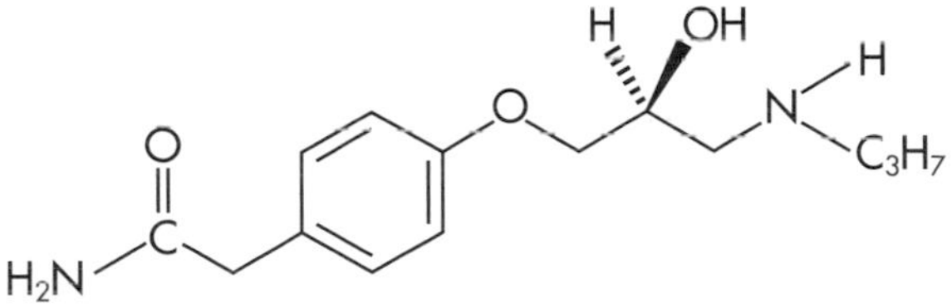

Figure 2.13 The structure of atenolol.

A 5 mL sample of plasma (pH 7.4) taken from a patient being treated with atenolol was extracted with 2 × 5 mL aliquots of ether. The ether layers were combined and evaporated to dryness and the residue was reconstituted in 5 mL of methanol. The concentration of atenolol in the methanol was found to be 0.604 μg mL^{-1}.

Calculate the original concentration of atenolol in the plasma sample and the percentage of the drug extracted.

How might the extraction procedure be altered to improve the percentage of the drug removed?

(Answers to problems can be found on pp. 215–217.)

3

Physicochemical properties of drugs

As has been stated before, most of the drugs used in medicine behave in solution as weak acids, weak bases, or sometimes as both weak acids and weak bases. In this chapter we will explore the reasons why drugs behave as acids or bases and what effects ionisation has on the properties of the drug, and develop strategies to separate mixtures of drugs on the basis of changes in their solubility in various solvents.

The most important thing to realise about acidic and basic drugs is that values of pK_a and pK_b quoted in the literature tell you *absolutely nothing* about whether the drug in question is an acid or a base. The pK_a and pK_b values give information about the strength of acids and bases; they tell you the pH at which 50% of the drug is ionised, but they do not tell you whether a drug behaves as an acid or a base in solution. Amines, for example are basic and have pK_a values of approximately 9, while phenols are acidic and typically have pK_a values of around 10. *The only sure way to know whether a drug is acidic or basic is to learn the functional groups that confer acidity and basicity on a molecule.* This should be done even if it means learning the names of the functional groups the way you learned multiplication tables at primary school. There are only a few to learn and the important examples are listed below along with some common drugs.

Carboxylic acids

According to the Brønsted–Lowry definition, an acid is a substance that ionises to donate protons to its surroundings. In aqueous solution this is represented as

$$HA + H_2O \rightleftharpoons H_3O^+ + A^- \tag{3.1}$$

where HA is the acid, water accepts the proton and acts as a base, H_3O^+ is a solvated proton, sometimes called the conjugate acid of the base and A^- is the anion of the acid. The equilibrium constant for this reaction is the acid dissociation constant, K_a and is expressed mathematically as

$$K_a = \frac{[H_3O^+][A^-]}{HA} \tag{3.2}$$

(taking $[H_2O]$ to be effectively constant for dilute solutions).

From equation (3.2) it can be seen that since K_a is a simple ratio, the higher the numerical value of K_a the stronger will be the acid. As stated in Chapter 1, however, the strength of most acids (and bases) is expressed by the term pK_a, where

$$pK_a = -\log_{10} K_a \tag{3.3}$$

Since pK_a is the negative logarithm of K_a, it follows that the *lower* the value of pK_a the *stronger* will be the acid and that on a log scale a difference of one unit in pK_a reflects a tenfold difference in acid strength.

The most commonly occurring functional group confering acidity on drug molecules is the carboxyl group, which ionises as shown in Figure 3.1. The anion formed by ionisation of the acid is stabilised by the process of *resonance*. Neither of the two conventional structures ([a] and [b]) of the carboxylate anion shown in Figure 3.2 is correct. A C=O double bond is much shorter than a C—O single bond (due to sideways repulsion of the electrons in the bond), yet when the carbon–oxygen bond lengths of the carboxylate anion are measured (e.g. by X-ray diffraction) they are found to be precisely the same length – shorter than a single bond and longer than a double bond. It would also be wrong to say that the actual structure of the carboxylate anion is a single structure rapidly interchanging between [a] and [b]. Structures [a] and [b] represent extremes of the actual structure. It is better to say the actual structure of the anion is a single, symmetrical structure inter-mediate between [a] and [b] in which the charge is delocalised (distri-buted) around the carboxylate group. This effect is called *resonance* and is invoked when not all of the observed properties of a compound can be explained or represented by conventional structures. The carboxylate anion is said to be a *resonance hybrid* and [a] and [b] are *canonical forms* that contribute to it. The resonance hybrid is generally a more

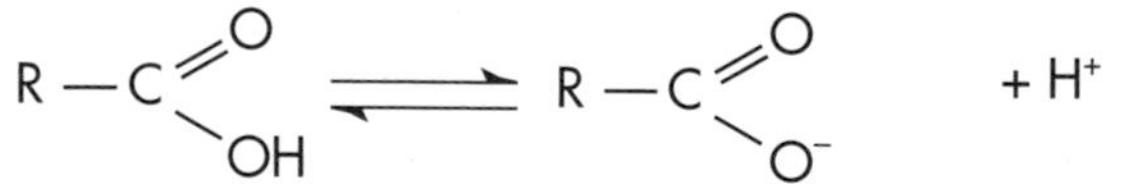

Figure 3.1   The ionisation of a carboxylic acid.

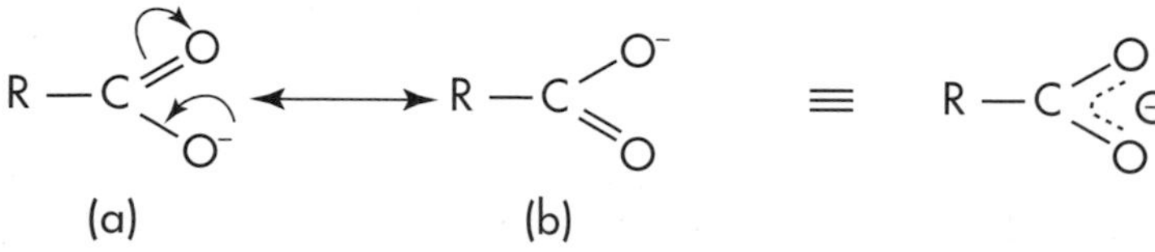

Figure 3.2   Resonance stabilisation of the carboxylate anion.

stable structure than either of the canonical forms, which means it is more likely to exist, which is another way of saying the carboxylic acid is more likely to ionise, which means it is a stronger acid.

The effect of resonance may be seen when the acidity of a simple carboxylic acid such as acetic acid is compared with the acidity of an alcohol such as ethanol. Both compounds can ionise to liberate a proton, but while the anion formed on ionisation of acetic acid is resonance-stabilised, the ethoxide anion formed on ionisation of ethanol is not so stabilised and the negative charge resides wholly on the oxygen atom (see Figure 3.3).

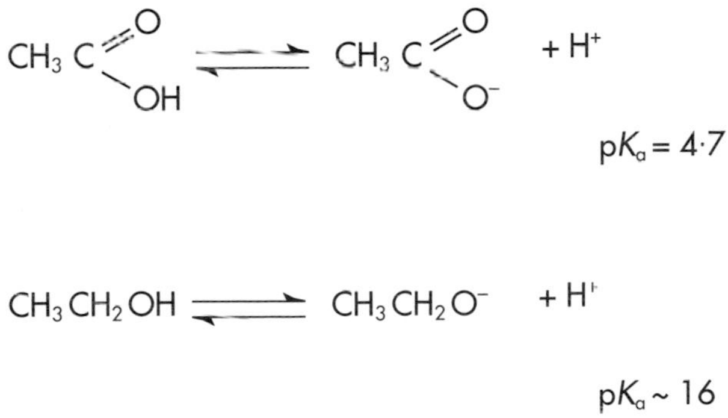

$$CH_3\,C\overset{\displaystyle O}{\underset{\displaystyle OH}{\Big<}} \rightleftharpoons CH_3\,C\overset{\displaystyle O}{\underset{\displaystyle O^-}{\Big<}} + H^+$$

$$pK_a = 4{\cdot}7$$

$$CH_3\,CH_2\,OH \rightleftharpoons CH_3\,CH_2\,O^- + H^+$$

$$pK_a \sim 16$$

Figure 3.3 The ionisations of acetic acid and ethanol.

The pK_a of acetic acid is 4.7 while the pK_a of ethanol is approximately 16. This means that acetic acid is almost a hundred thousand million (or 10^{11}) times more acidic than ethanol. Alcohols are much weaker acids than water and in biological systems are considered to be neutral. To bring about the ionisation of an alcohol requires the use of a very strong base such as metallic sodium.

A number of commonly used drugs are carboxylic acid derivatives. These include aspirin (pK_a 3.5), the anticancer compound methotrexate (pK_a 3.8, 4.8 and 5.6) and the diuretic etacrynic acid (pK_a 3.5). The structures of these compounds are shown in Figure 3.4.

Knowledge of the pK_a value of a drug and the approximate rule of thumb introduced in Chapter 1 allows a prediction of the extent to which each of these drugs is ionised at the pH of human blood (7.4). For aspirin and etacrynic acid with pK_a values of 3.5, the answer is that 99.99% of a given dose of drug will be ionised at the pH of blood or intracellular fluid. For methotrexate the answer will be slightly less, but still greater than 99%. This strongly suggests that these drugs are

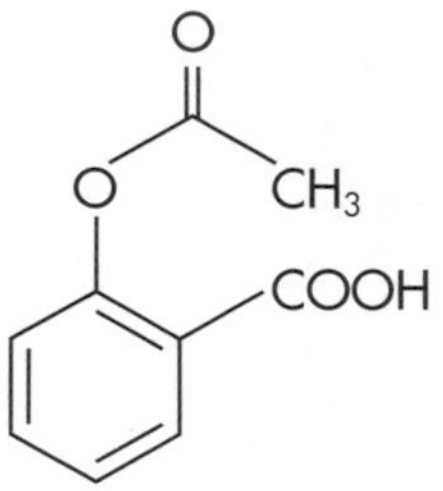

Aspirin 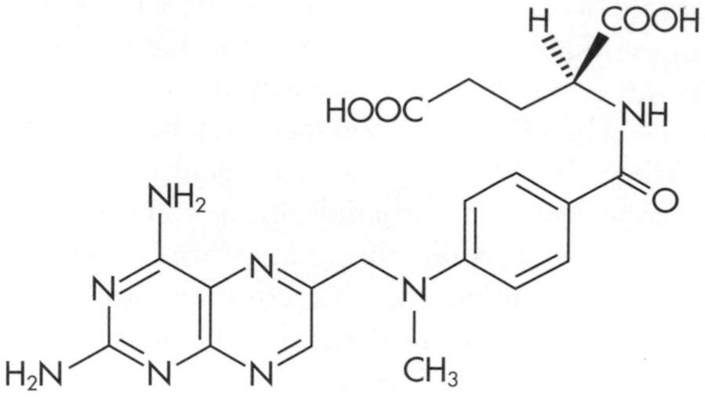   Methotrexate

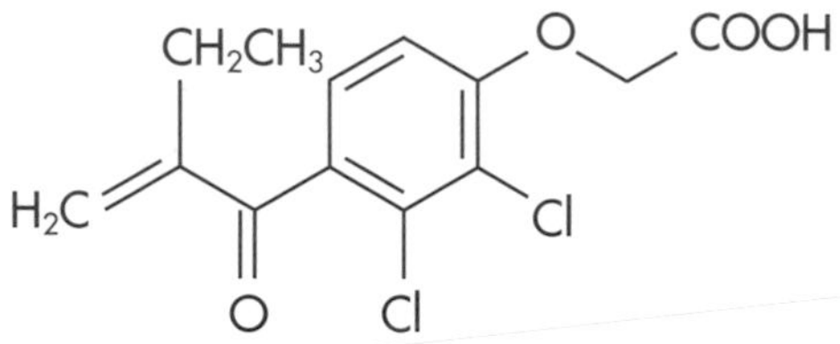

Etacrynic acid

Figure 3.4 The structures of aspirin, methotrexate and etacrynic acid.

pharmacologically active as the anion, and interact with their individual receptors in the ionic form. This conclusion has been reached without considering the detailed three-dimensional structure of each drug's receptor molecule, merely by applying knowledge of the pK_a and an appreciation of the extent to which drugs ionise in solution. Deductions of this type form the basis of *medicinal chemistry*, the science of rational drug design.

Phenols

Another commonly encountered acidic functional group found in drug molecules is phenol, or hydroxybenzene. Phenols are weak acids that liberate protons to give the phenoxide anion. This anion is resonance-stabilised and four canonical forms may be drawn (see Figure 3.5).

As with carboxylic acids, the effect of resonance is to distribute the negative charge around the anion, rather than have it concentrated on

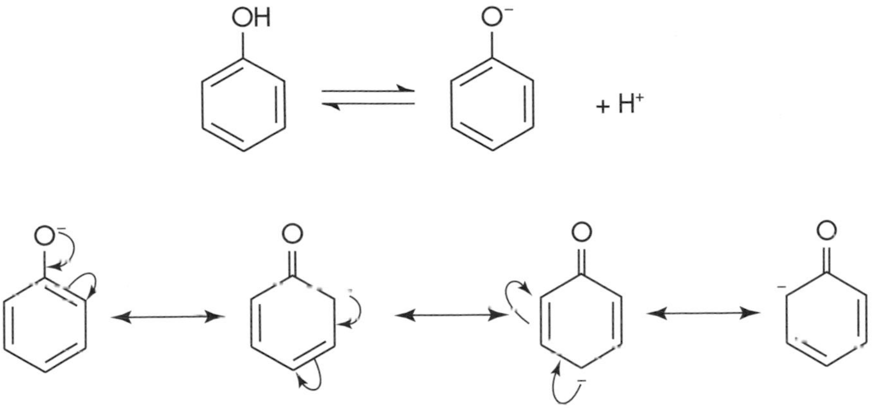

Figure 3.5 Resonance stabilisation of the phenoxide anion.

the oxygen atom. Phenols have pK_a values of approximately 10, which means they are about a million times less acidic than carboxylic acids but are about a million times more acidic than simple alcohols. Phenols are also weaker acids than carbonic acid (H_2CO_3), which means that they do not react with sodium bicarbonate (cf. carboxylic acids) and may be precipitated from solution of the phenoxide by saturation with carbon dioxide.

A number of common drugs contain the phenol functional group. These include paracetamol (pK_a 9.5), morphine (pK_a 9.9) and levothyroxine (thyroxine) (pK_a 10). Since these phenolic drugs are 50% ionised when the pH equals their pK_a, it follows from the 'rule of thumb' introduced in Chapter 1 that they will only ionise to approximately 1% at the pH of blood (7.4). See Figure 3.6.

Warfarin

Warfarin is an anticoagulant that inhibits the clotting action of blood through an action on vitamin K-derived clotting factors. It is commonly prescribed to elderly patients who suffer from deep-vein thrombosis or pulmonary embolism. Warfarin is used in the UK as the sodium salt, which strongly suggests that the drug is acidic, though the presence of the acidic hydrogen may not be immediately apparent. The acidic hydrogen (drawn in bold in Figure 3.7) is located between two electron-withdrawing carbonyl groups. Upon ionisation, the negative charge can be delocalised onto each of the electronegative oxygen atoms of the dicarbonyl group to yield a resonance-stabilised anion. This enhanced

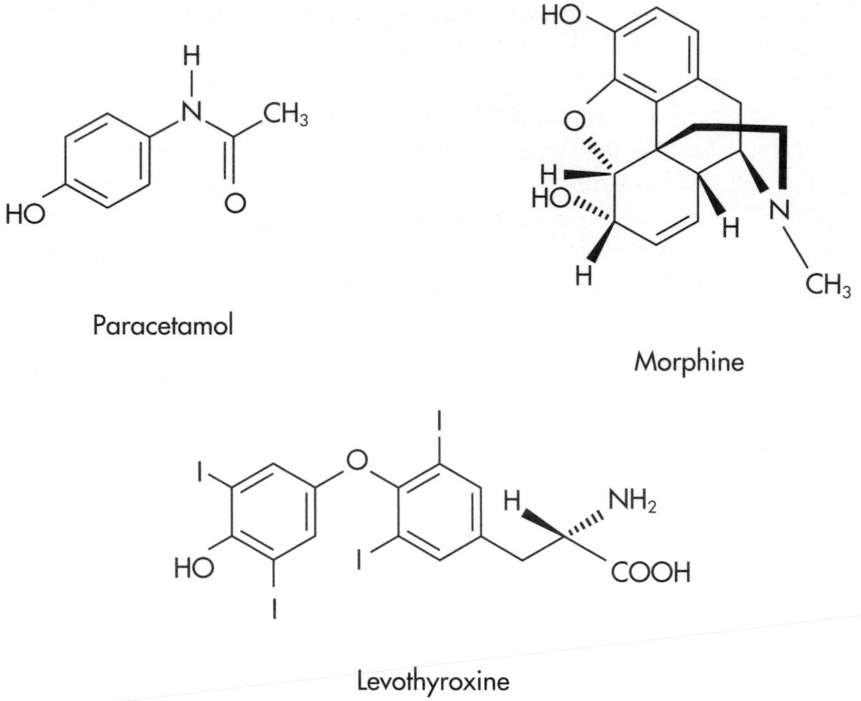

Paracetamol

Morphine

Levothyroxine

Figure 3.6 The structures of paracetamol, morphine and levothyroxine.

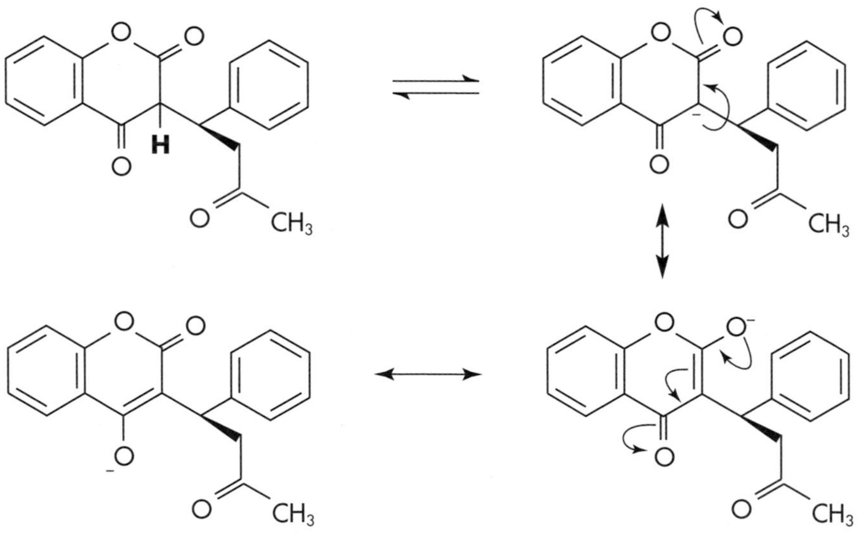

Figure 3.7 The ionisation of warfarin.

stability of the anion allows warfarin to lose a proton and renders the drug acidic with a pK_a of 5.0. Warfarin in the free acid form is not very soluble in water and is therefore always administered (and is official in the British Pharmacopoeia) as the sodium salt.

Warfarin is an interesting compound in that, in addition to ionising, it exhibits keto–enol *tautomerism*. This means that warfarin exists in two constitutional isomeric forms (tautomers) that are in equilibrium with each other, although one of the forms is usually present to a much higher degree than the other. (See Figure 3.8.)

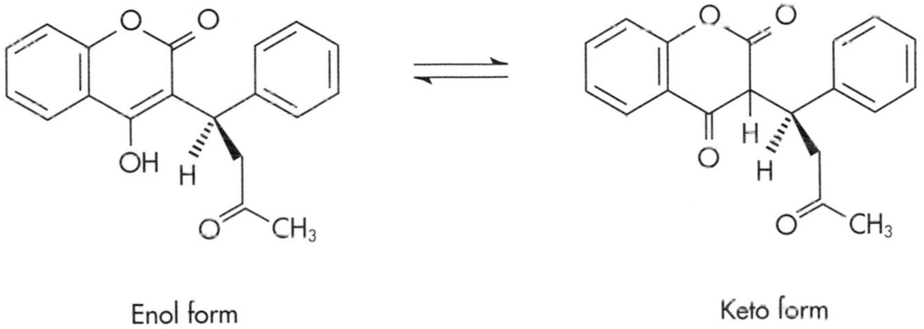

Enol form   Keto form

Figure 3.8 The tautomerism of warfarin.

It is important not to confuse the properties of tautomerism and resonance. They are quite different effects and the differences between them are summarised in Table 3.1. Although the enol form of warfarin is present to a very small extent, it is acceptable to consider the ionisation of the compound in terms of the enol, and this is shown in Figure 3.9.

Table 3.1 Comparison of resonance and tautomerism

Resonance forms of a drug[a]	Tautomeric forms of a drug[b]
Same compound	Different compounds
Differ only in position of *electrons*	Differ in position of *atoms* (usually hydrogen)
Each canonical form contributes to a single resonance structure	Each form exists in equilibrium
Canonical forms cannot be isolated	Each tautomer may be isolated

[a] Represented by a double-headed arrow ↔.
[b] Represented by an equilibrium arrow ⇌.

There is a popular misconception that, because amines are basic and amines contain a nitrogen atom, then all drugs that contain nitrogen

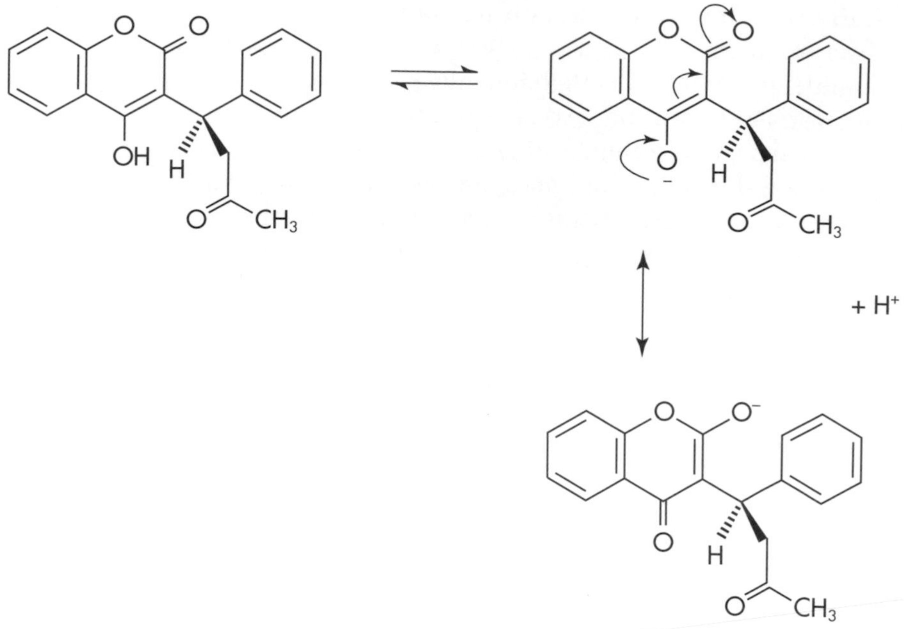

Figure 3.9   The ionisation of the enol form of warfarin.

will be basic. This is not true, as a moment's thought will confirm. Amides contain nitrogen and are neutral, and quite a few drugs containing nitrogen atoms are actually acidic. Compounds are basic only if the lone pair of electrons on the nitrogen is available for reaction with protons. In the case of amides, the carbon–nitrogen bond has significant double-bond character due to resonance, as shown in Figure 3.10.

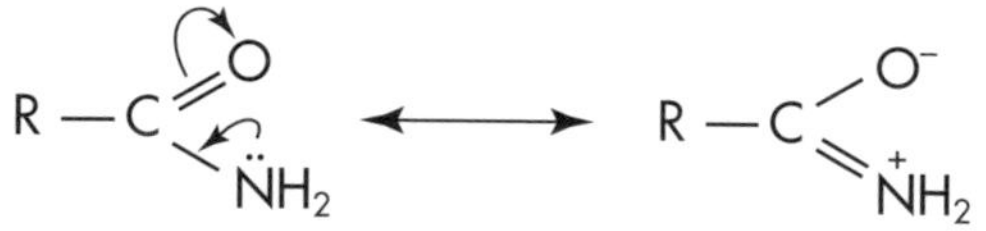

Figure 3.10   Resonance effects of the amide group.

The lone pair of electrons on the nitrogen of some drug molecules can be completely unavailable for reaction with protons. Drugs of this type are so weakly basic that they actually behave as *acids* in solution. This effect can be illustrated by considering the compounds below.

Phenylbutazone

Phenylbutazone is a non-steroidal anti-inflammatory drug (or NSAID) that exerts its anti-inflammatory action through inhibition of the enzyme cyclo-oxygenase and inhibition of the production of inflammatory mediators such as prostaglandins. Phenylbutazone, despite containing nitrogen, is a weak acid with a pK_a of 4.4. The acidic hydrogen is on the 4-position of the pyrazolidinedione ring and upon ionisation the negative charge is delocalised onto the adjacent carbonyl groups in a similar manner to that in warfarin (pK_a 5.0). See Figure 3.11.

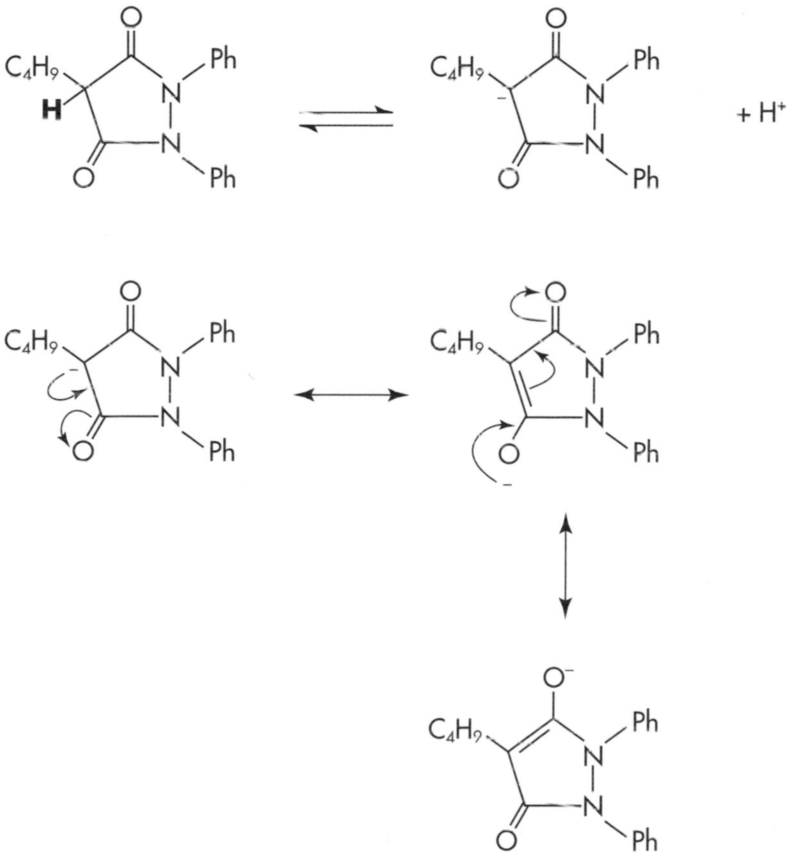

Figure 3.11   The ionisation of phenylbutazone.

Indometacin

Indometacin is another NSAID with a similar mode of action to that of phenylbutazone. Indometacin is acidic due to ionisation of the carboxylic acid group. The nitrogen atom in indometacin is present as an amide and is essentially neutral. See Figure 3.12.

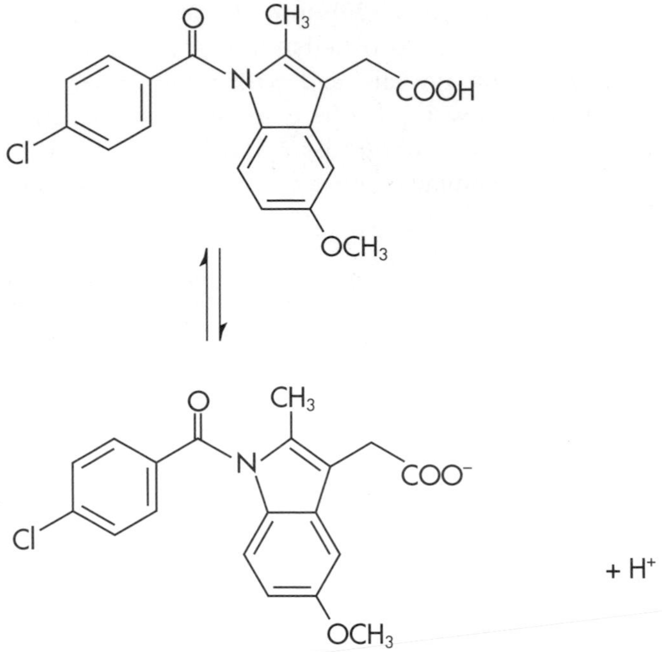

Figure 3.12 The ionisation of indometacin.

Barbiturates

Barbiturates are cyclic imides used as hypnotics and (in the case of phenobarbital) as anticonvulsants. They are all derivatives of barbituric acid (which is not pharmacologically active) and differ only in their substituents on the 5-position of the ring. Barbiturates contain nitrogen atoms, but the lone pair on the nitrogen is not available for reaction with protons, so barbiturates are not basic. Instead, they behave as weak acids in solution (dibasic actually, though the second ionisation is very weak); the negative charge formed on ionisation delocalises around the two adjacent carbonyl groups in a manner similar to that in warfarin. The pK_a values for barbiturates are typically 7–8 for the first ionisation and approximately 11–12 for the second, although the drugs are usually administered in the form of the sodium salt to increase water solubility. The first ionisation of a barbiturate is shown in Figure 3.13.

The sulfur analogue of pentobarbital, called thiopental (Figure 3.14), is widely used in operating theatres for the induction of general anaesthesia. Thiobarbiturates of this type have a much higher partition coefficient than the oxobarbiturates used as hypnotics (see Chapter 2). As a result, thiopental, when administered intravenously to

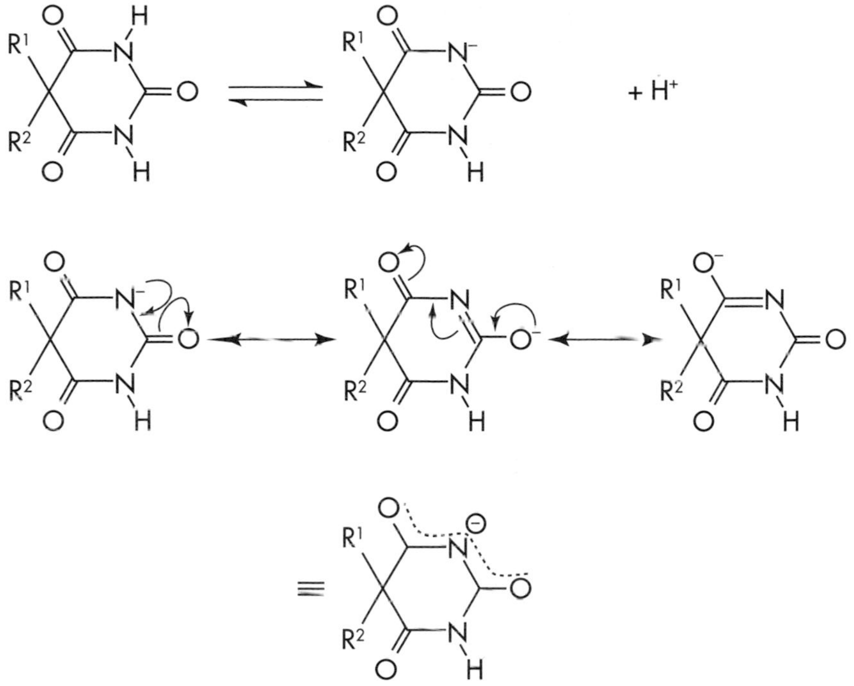

Figure 3.13 The ionisation of a barbiturate.

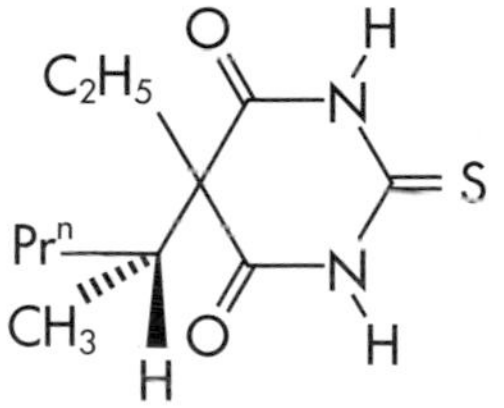

Figure 3.14 The structure of thiopental.

a vein in the back of the hand, can induce unconsciousness in a matter of seconds that lasts for several minutes. This is sufficient time for the anaesthetist to introduce an airway to the patient and commence general anaesthesia.

Phenytoin

Phenytoin is an anticonvulsant widely used in the treatment of epilepsy. The properties of phenytoin resemble those of barbiturates. It is a cyclic imide with a pK_a of 8.3. The anion is stabilised by resonance of the negative charge onto the carbonyl oxygens and the drug is usually administered as the sodium salt to increase water solubility. See Figure 3.15.

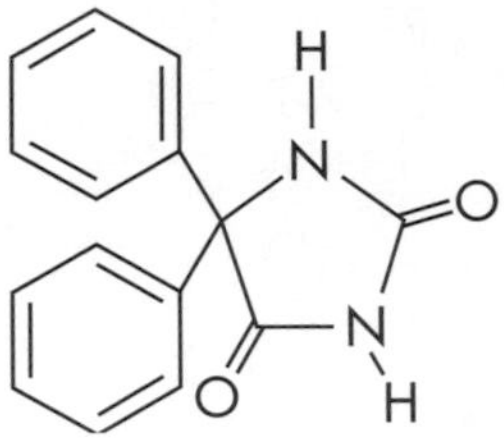

Figure 3.15 The structure of phenytoin.

Phenytoin and barbiturates display tautomerism of the imine–imide type, as shown in Figure 3.16. The predominant tautomer is the imide form, although some older textbooks list the structure of the drug as the minor tautomer.

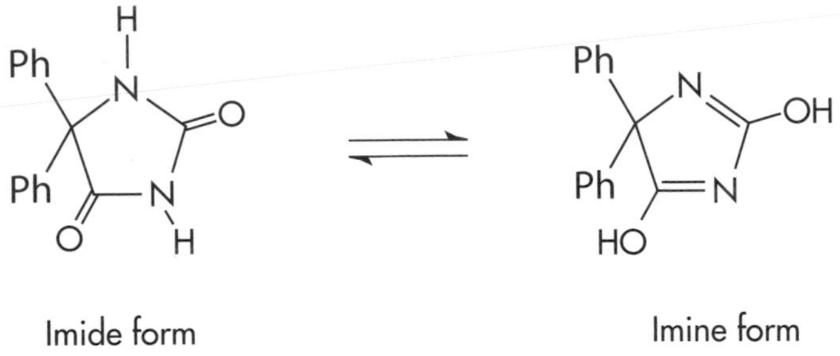

Imide form   Imine form

Figure 3.16 The tautomerism of phenytoin.

Sulfonamides

Sulfonamides are a class of antibacterial compounds, all of which contain the sulfonamido group $-SO_2NH$. Although they were widely used in the past, their use has decreased in recent years with the advent of newer antibiotics such as penicillins and cephalosporins.

Sulfonamides are all weakly acidic (pK_a approximately 5–8) due to the powerful electron-withdrawing effect of the $-SO_2-$ substituent and stabilisation of the resulting anion by resonance. Sulfonamides are usually administered in the form of the sodium salt to increase their water solubility. The ionisation of a sulfonamide is shown in Figure 3.17.

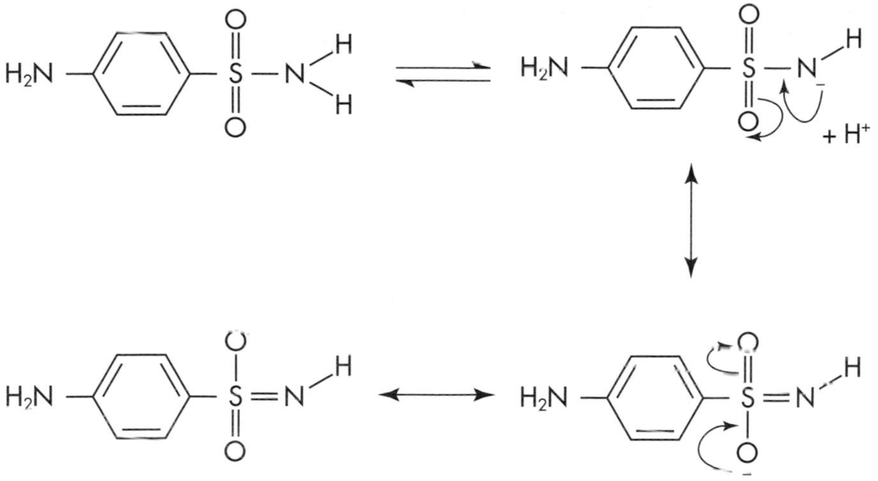

Figure 3.17   The ionisation of a sulfonamide.

Basic drugs

The Brønsted–Lowry definition of a base is an acceptor of protons. Pharmaceutical and biological sciences are concerned mainly with the behaviour of drugs in aqueous systems. Under these conditions, drugs will behave as bases only if they contain *a nitrogen atom with a lone pair of electrons available for reaction with protons*. The major class of compound to work in this way is the amines. An amine in aqueous solution will react with water to release hydroxide ions (OH⁻) as shown in equation (3.4).

$$R_3N + H_2O \rightleftharpoons R_3NH^+ + OH^- \tag{3.4}$$

Water donates the proton and functions as an acid in this reaction. The equilibrium constant for this reaction is defined as K_b and the greater the value of K_b the stronger will be the base.

$$K_b = \frac{[R_3NH^+][OH^-]}{[R_3N]} \tag{3.5}$$

However, as was discussed in Chapter 1, most of the pharmaceutical literature refers to the strength of bases in terms of the pK_a of the conjugate acid of the base. In this case, *the higher the value of pK_a the stronger is the base.*

Basic drugs are usually administered as their water-soluble salts (generally the hydrochloride). Care must be taken not to co-administer anything that will raise the pH of the hydrochloride salt solution in case precipitation of the less water-soluble free base occurs.

The key point to remember about basicity of amines is the availability of the lone pair of electrons on the nitrogen atom. If the lone pair is involved in interactions elsewhere in the molecule, then the amine will not be basic. This can be illustrated by consideration of the basicity of the local anaesthetic procaine. See Figure 3.18. The nitrogen of the diethylamino moiety is present in a tertiary amine. The lone pair of electrons is concentrated on the nitrogen atom and is available to accept a proton. This means the aliphatic nitrogen can ionise at the pH of human plasma (pH 7.4) to form the mono-cation of procaine. Conversely, the lone pair of electrons on the amino group attached to the benzene ring is less available for reaction with protons due to delocalisation into the ring. This delocalisation increases the electron density of the *ortho* and *para* carbon atoms and means that the Ar-NH$_2$ group does not ionise at the pH of blood.

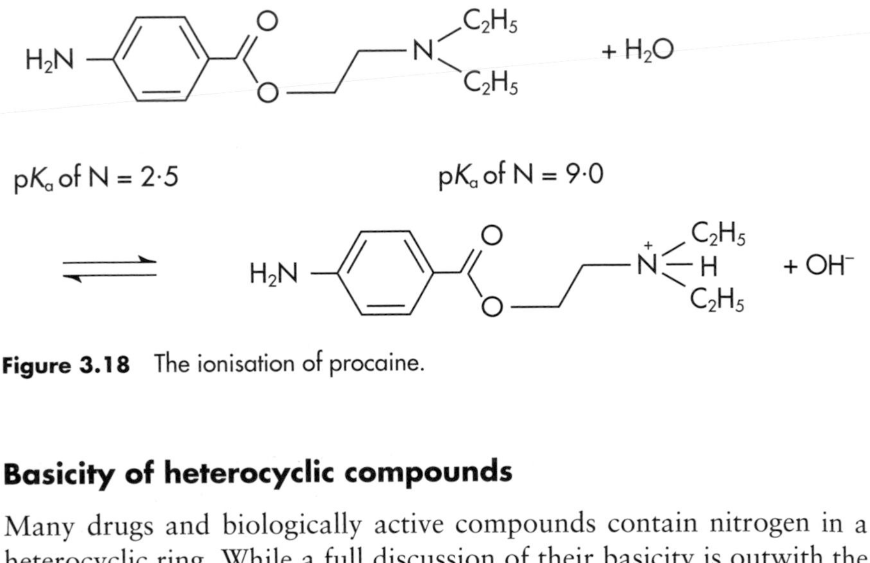

pK$_a$ of N = 2·5   pK$_a$ of N = 9·0

Figure 3.18 The ionisation of procaine.

Basicity of heterocyclic compounds

Many drugs and biologically active compounds contain nitrogen in a heterocyclic ring. While a full discussion of their basicity is outwith the scope of this book, a brief summary of factors influencing basicity will be considered.

In *aliphatic heterocyclic compounds*, the nitrogen atom is part of a saturated heterocyclic ring and the lone pair of electrons is available for reaction with protons (e.g. piperidine, Figure 3.19). Compounds of this type are similar in base strength to their open-chain aliphatic counterparts with typical pK$_a$ values of 8–9.

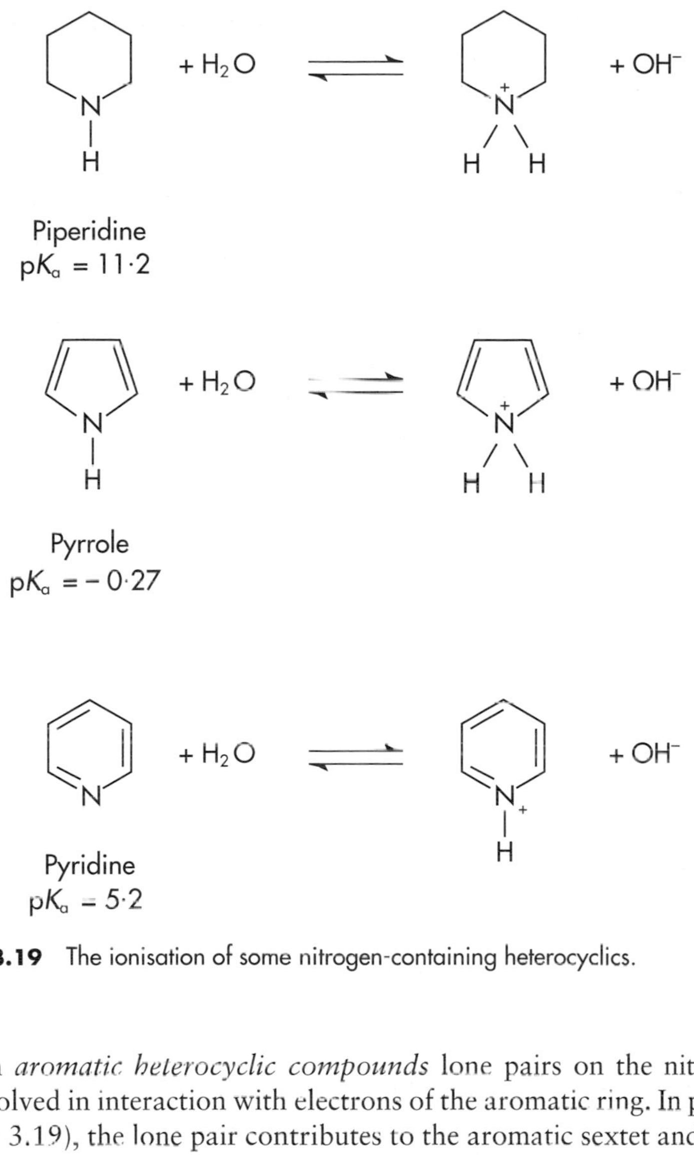

Piperidine
$pK_a = 11\cdot2$

Pyrrole
$pK_a = -0\cdot27$

Pyridine
$pK_a = 5\cdot2$

Figure 3.19 The ionisation of some nitrogen-containing heterocyclics.

In *aromatic heterocyclic compounds* lone pairs on the nitrogens are involved in interaction with electrons of the aromatic ring. In pyrrole (Figure 3.19), the lone pair contributes to the aromatic sextet and is not available for reaction with protons. As a result, pyrrole is a very weak base with a pK_a value so low that it is a negative number.

The six-membered nitrogen heterocycle pyridine (Figure 3.19) is also a weak base. In the case of pyridine, however, only one electron from the nitrogen contributes to the aromatic sextet. This leaves an unshared pair of electrons, which can accept a proton, so that pyridine is measurably basic with a pK_a value of 5.2. This value is similar to that found in aromatic amines such as aniline or aminobenzene.

Separation of mixtures

It is often the case that pharmaceutical and/or chemical procedures give rise to mixtures of chemicals. These could arise as a result of incomplete chemical reaction, as in the case of side-reactions and by-products, or when drugs have to be isolated from complex mixtures of chemicals (e.g. isolation of a drug metabolite from a blood or urine sample). A knowledge of the acidity and basicity of drugs is essential if efficient separation is to be achieved. When a drug molecule ionises, the solubility profile of the compound changes dramatically. Free acids and bases when they are unionised tend to dissolve well in non-polar organic solvents such as diethyl ether, chloroform or ethyl acetate. Upon ionisation, the acid will form an anion and the base will form a conjugate acid. These will both be more soluble in aqueous solvents such as water or buffer. This means that acidic drugs are soluble in organic solvents at low pH (when they are primarily unionised) and soluble in polar solvents at high pH. Bases, conversely, are soluble in organic solvents when the pH is high (and the base is unionised) and are water soluble at low values of pH.

Solubility differences of this type allow the separation of some quite complex mixtures to be carried out easily and quickly in the laboratory. All that is needed is a pair of immiscible solvents, a separating funnel and an understanding of the effects of pH on the solubility of drugs. An example of this type of separation is shown below.

Tutorial examples

Q *1   An 'over-the-counter' analgesic called APC Tablets contains aspirin, paracetamol and codeine. An extract of these tablets was dissolved in toluene (methylbenzene) and filtered to remove insoluble solids. Devise a separation scheme to isolate all three drugs in a pure form.*

A 1   The structures and pK_a values of the three drugs are shown in Figure 3.20.

Aspirin and paracetamol are both acidic compounds, while codeine is a weak base. If a student cannot correctly identify whether the drugs in question are acids or bases, the whole question will be wrong and misery will surely follow. There is no easy way to do this other than to learn (parrot fashion if necessary) the functional groups that cause a drug to function as an acid or a base.

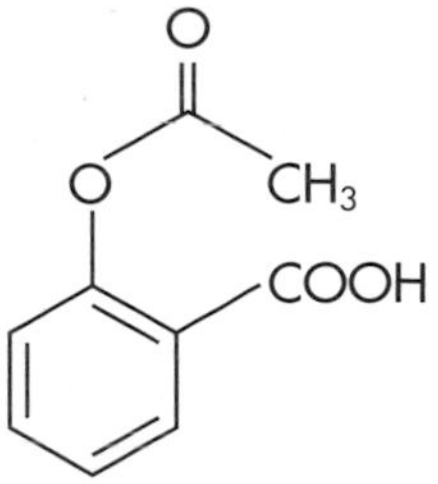

Aspirin pK_a = 2·5

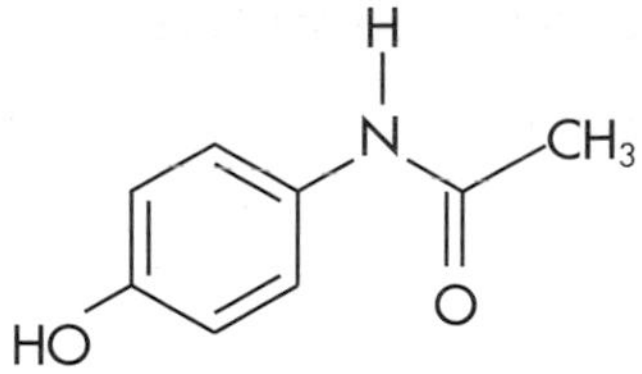

Paracetamol pK_a = 9·5

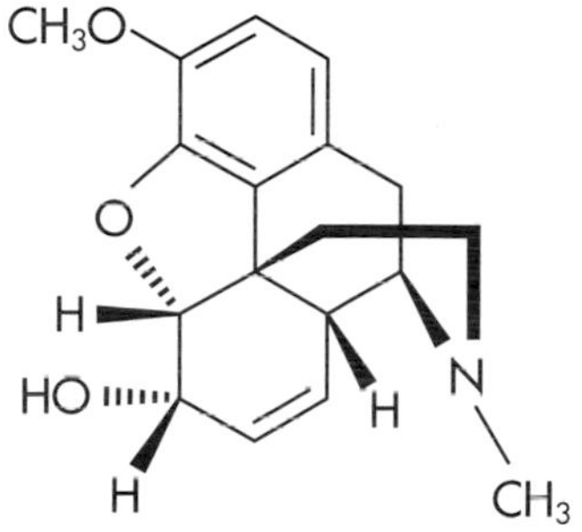

Codeine pK_a = 8·2

Figure 3.20 The structures and pK_a of aspirin, paracetamol and codeine.

All three drugs will be soluble in toluene in their unionised form. The separation strategy is to ionise the drugs sequentially and remove them in the aqueous phase, whereupon back extraction into an organic solvent will yield the (hopefully) pure compounds.

Addition of dilute hydrochloric acid will ionise the codeine and form codeine hydrochloride. This salt will be water soluble and will partition into the aqueous (lower) phase. Removal of the aqueous phase and addition of fresh organic solvent and a strong base (such as sodium hydroxide) will liberate codeine base in the organic phase. Evaporation of the volatile solvent yields pure codeine.

Aspirin is a carboxylic acid derivative, while paracetamol is a substituted phenol. Addition of a strong base (e.g. sodium hydroxide) would result in ionisation of both acids. To separate the acids successfully, a discriminating base must therefore be used, which is formed from an acid intermediate in strength between carboxylic acids and phenols. Such an acid is carbonic acid (H_2CO_3) and addition of sodium bicarbonate solution will result in ionisation of the aspirin as the sodium salt. This salt will be water soluble and may be removed in the lower phase. Addition of fresh organic solvent and dilute hydrochloric acid solution will yield aspirin as free acid.

The remaining drug, paracetamol, may be isolated by simple evaporation of the toluene or extracted into aqueous solvent by addition of a strong base such as sodium hydroxide solution.

The separation is shown schematically in Figure 3.21.

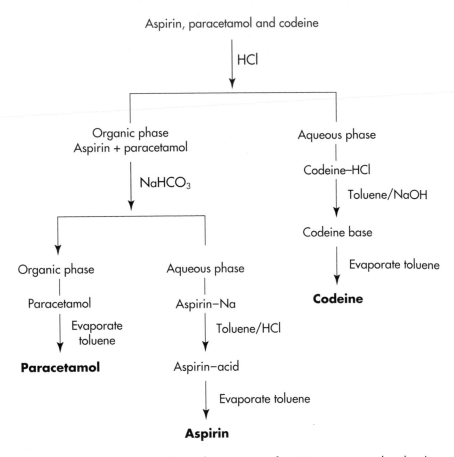

Figure 3.21 A separation scheme for a mixture of aspirin, paracetamol and codeine.

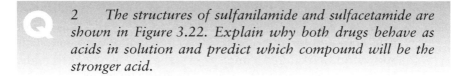

> 2   *The structures of sulfanilamide and sulfacetamide are shown in Figure 3.22. Explain why both drugs behave as acids in solution and predict which compound will be the stronger acid.*

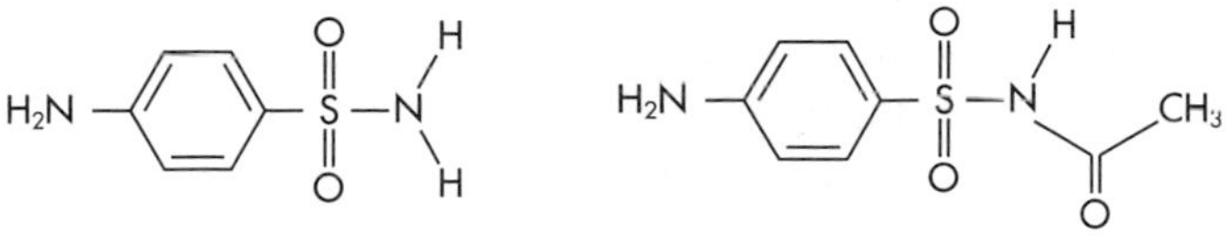

Sulfanilamide   Sulfacetamide

Figure 3.22   The structure of sulfanilamide and sulfacetamide.

2   Both drugs are sulfonamides and ionise with the release of a proton. The anion formed is stabilised by resonance as discussed previously. The pK_a value for sulfanilamide is 10.4, while the pK_a of sulfacetamide is 5.4. Clearly, since the value of pK_a is lower, sulfacetamide is a much stronger acid than sul-

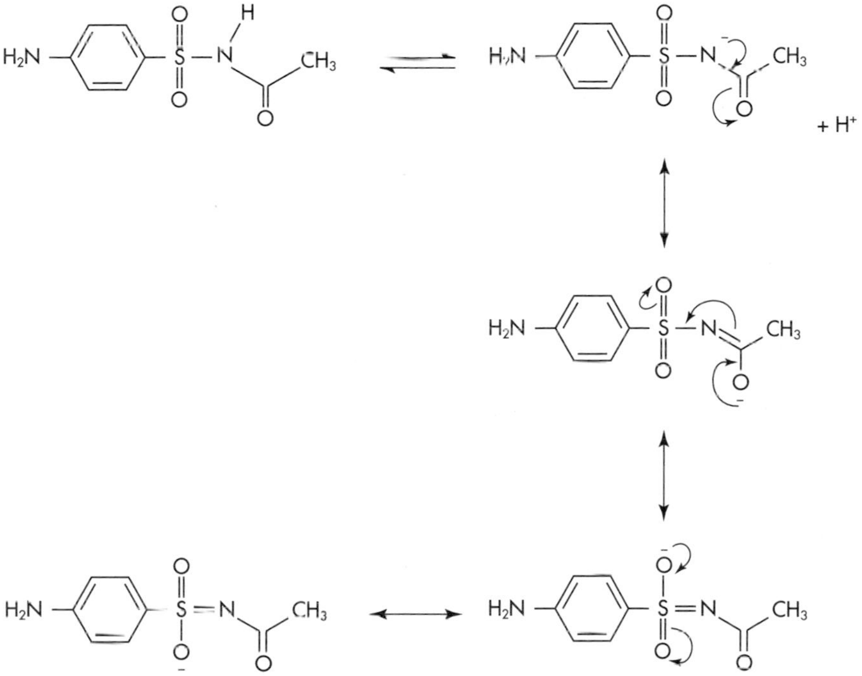

Figure 3.23   Resonance effects in sulfacetamide.

fanilamide (five units difference on a log scale = 100 000 times stronger). This difference in acidity is caused by the presence of a carbonyl group adjacent to the sulfonamido hydrogen. This allows additional resonance to take place in sulfacetamide. Upon ionisation, the negative charge on the anion can delocalise onto the carbonyl oxygen as shown in Figure 3.23. This delocalisation further stabilises the anion and is in addition to the normal resonance present in the sulfonamido-group.

Problems

Q3.1   Co-trimoxazole tablets contain sulfamethoxazole and trimethoprim and are used in the treatment of chest and urinary tract infections. Classify sulfamethoxazole and trimethoprim as acidic, basic or neutral and hence describe how you could separate a mixture of the two drugs in the laboratory using simple glassware and reagents. See Figure 3.24.

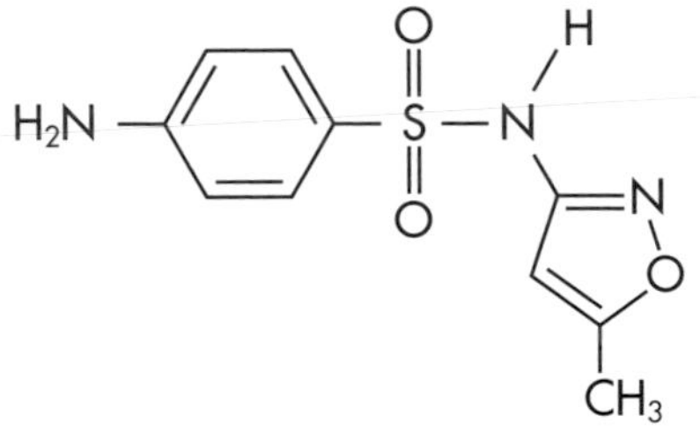

Sulfamethoxazole

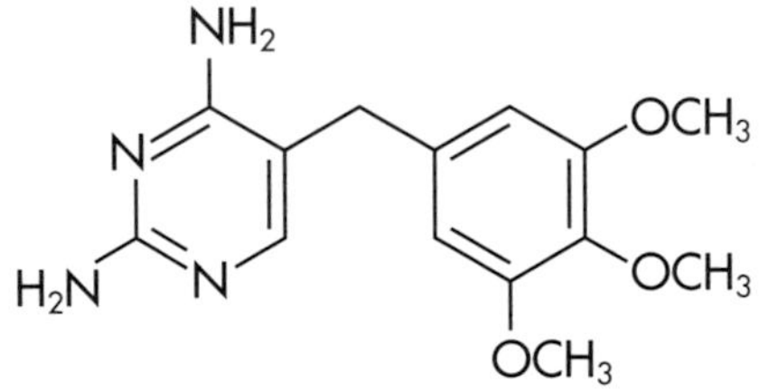

Trimethoprim

Figure 3.24   The structure of sulfamethoxazole and trimethoprim.

Q3.2 Refer to the structures numbered 1 to 6 in Figure 3.25. In each case select the form of the drug that predominates in human plasma at pH 7.4:

(a) Mono-cation
(b) Di-cation
(c) Mono-anion
(d) Di-anion
(e) Neutral molecule

1. 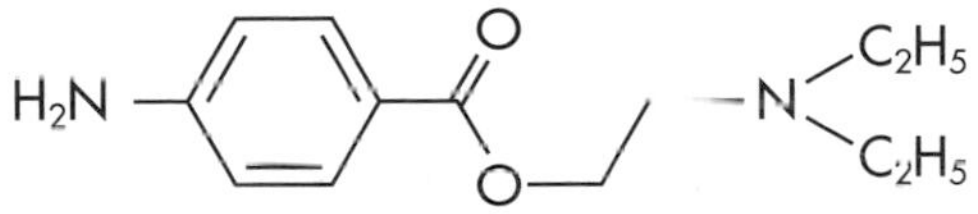

2. 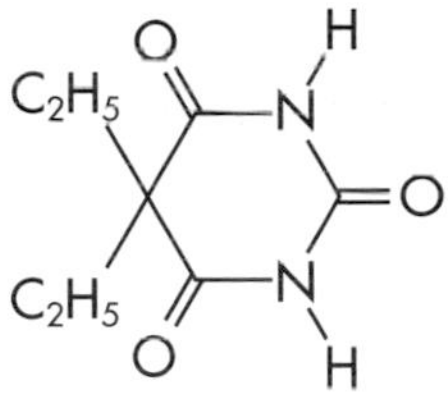

3. 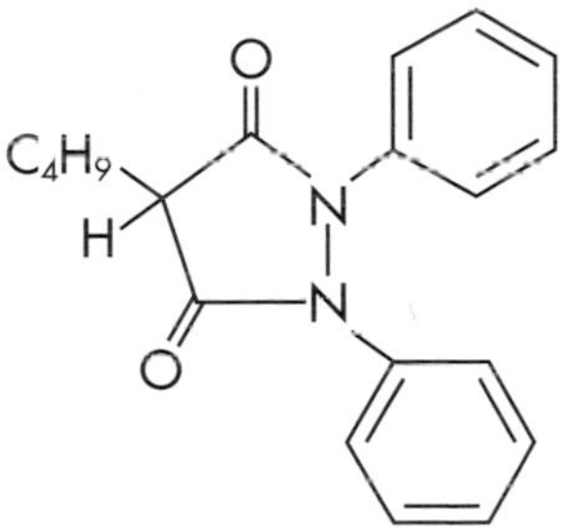

4. 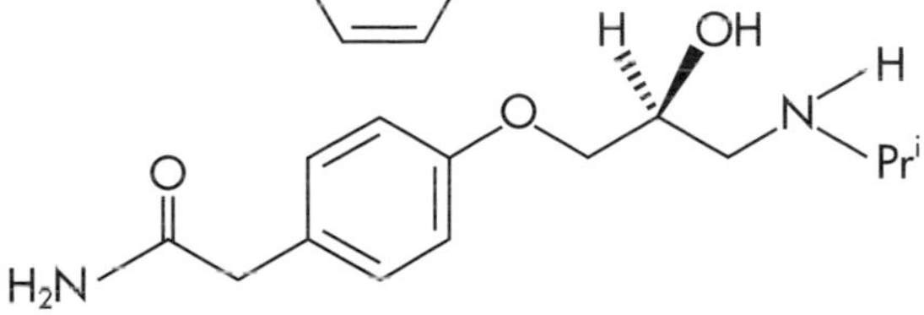

5. CH_3CH_2OH

6. 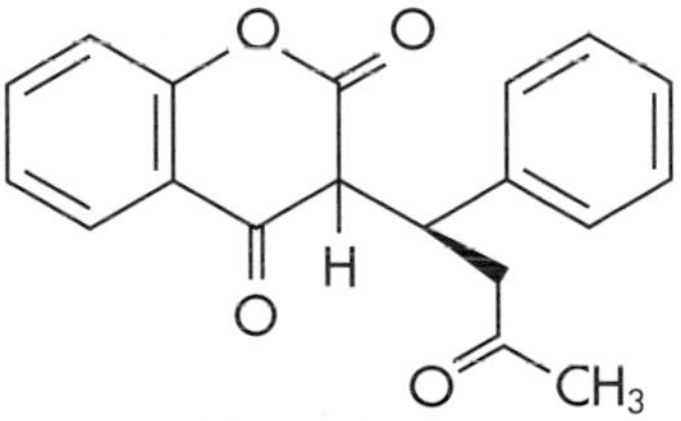

Figure 3.25 Structures of drugs.

Q3.3 The structure of nicotine is shown in Figure 3.26. Classify nicotine as acidic, basic or neutral, draw the structure of the form of nicotine that will predominate at plasma pH, and suggest the form of nicotine that is active pharmacologically.

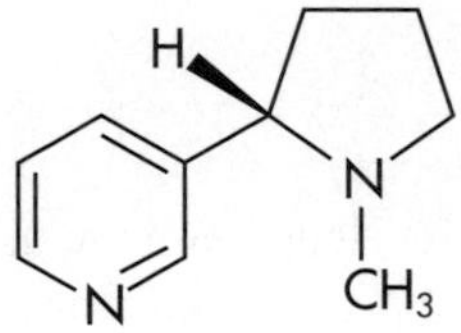

Figure 3.26 The structure of nicotine.

(Answers to problems can be found on pp. 217–219.)

4

Stereochemistry

In Chapter 3 the reasons why drugs behave as weak acids or weak bases were discussed and strategies were developed to exploit differences in physicochemical properties to separate components of a mixture. In this chapter, the three-dimensional shapes of molecules will be introduced and, in particular, the unusual geometry that arises around a carbon atom with four different substituents attached to it – an *asymmetric carbon atom*. The study of the three-dimensional shape of molecules is absolutely fundamental to a student's understanding of complex topics such as biochemistry, medicinal chemistry and drug design.

Chemical compounds that have the same molecular formula but different structural formulas are said to be *isomers* of each other. These constitutional isomers (or structural isomers) differ in their bonding sequence, i.e. their atoms are connected to each other in different ways. Stereoisomers have the same bonding sequence, but they differ in the orientation of their atoms in space. Stereoisomerism can be further divided into optical isomerism (*enantiomerism*) and *geometrical isomerism* (*cis–trans* isomerism). The relationships between the different types of isomerism are shown in Figure 4.1.

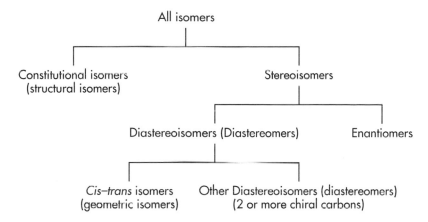

Figure 4.1 Different types of isomerism.

There are a number of atoms that display optical isomerism, including nitrogen and phosphorus, but the simplest case to consider, and the most commonly encountered in drugs, is that of an sp^3 hybridised carbon atom with four different substituents attached to it (Figure 4.2). A carbon like this is said to be *chiral* and to display the property of *chirality*. If the four substituents are different, a pair of non-superimposable mirror image forms can be drawn. These two isomers are called *enantiomers*. A chiral compound always has an enantiomer, whereas an achiral compound has a mirror image that is the same as the original molecule.

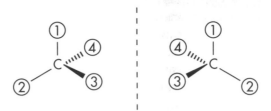

Figure 4.2   Chiral carbon atoms.

Enantiomers have identical or nearly identical physical properties unless a reagent or technique is used that is itself chiral. For example, the two enantiomers in Figure 4.2 will have the same boiling point, melting point, refractive index and density since these are bulk effects and cannot discriminate between the two enantiomers. Differences between enantiomers only become apparent when they interact with chiral reagents such as the active sites of enzymes or the chiral stationary phase of a HPLC column.

In the laboratory, the technique of *polarimetry* is used to distinguish between enantiomers and to measure the extent to which each enantiomer rotates the plane of plane-polarised light.

Polarimetry

Most of the light detected by our eyes is not polarised, that is the light waves vibrate randomly in all directions perpendicular to the direction of propagation of the wave. If normal light of this type is passed through a material that is itself chiral (e.g. the mineral Icelandic spar, or the compound, Polaroid, used in sunglasses) then the waves of light interact with the chiral material to produce light that is oscillating in only one plane. This light is called *plane-polarised light*. When plane-polarised light is passed through a solution containing an optically active substance, the chiral compound causes the plane of vibration of the light to rotate (the origin of the expression *optical activity*). If a second piece of chiral material fitted with a measuring protractor is now placed in the light path, the number of degrees of rotation can be measured and read off a calibrated scale. This is a description of an instrument called a polarimeter, which is used to measure the angle of rotation of plane-polarised light (Figure 4.3).

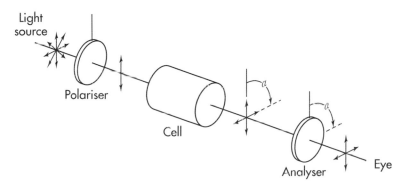

Figure 4.3 A diagram of a polarimeter.

The light source used in polarimetry is usually a sodium vapour lamp, which emits yellow light of a characteristic wavelength (the sodium D line, 589.3 nm). This light is polarised by a fixed filter (the polariser) and passed through a sample cell containing a solution of the optically active substance. The plane of the light is rotated by the chiral compound and emerges from the sample cell, whereupon it enters a second, movable filter (the analyser). This filter has a scale marked out in degrees and allows the operator to measure the angle between the two filters and hence the angle of rotation of the light, α. Once the angle of rotation has been measured the *specific optical rotation* $[\alpha]$ of the substance may be calculated.

$$[\alpha] = \frac{100\alpha}{lc} \tag{4.1}$$

where $[\alpha]$ = specific optical rotation, α = measured rotation in degrees, l = length of sample tube in decimetres (1 dm = 10 cm), c = concentration of sample in % w/v.

Values of $[\alpha]$ are quoted in British Pharmacopoeia (BP) monographs for chiral drugs and reagents and limits are set within which drugs of BP quality must comply. The specific optical rotation of a solid is always expressed with reference to a given solvent and concentration. The specific optical rotation of a liquid is obtained from equation (4.2). where d = relative density of the liquid.

$$[\alpha] = \frac{\alpha}{ld} \tag{4.2}$$

Compounds that rotate the plane of polarised light towards the right (clockwise) are called *dextrorotatory*, while compounds that rotate the plane to the left, or anticlockwise, are called *laevorotatory*. The direction of rotation is often specified by the symbols (+) for dextrorotatory and (−) for laevorotatory and the direction is considered with the operator facing the light source.

If a sample cell in a polarimeter contains equal amounts of the (+) and the (−) enantiomers, the angle of rotation due to one enantiomer will be equal and opposite to the angle due to the other and the net observed rotation will be zero. Such a mixture is called a *racemic mixture* or a *racemate* and is often encountered in the laboratory as a result of a non-chiral organic synthesis. The common synthesis of adrenaline (epinephrine), the 'fight or flight' hormone, yields a racemic mixture, which has precisely 50% of the biological activity of the natural hormone. Once the racemate is *resolved* into the two pure enantiomers, the (R)-(−)-adrenaline is found to be identical to the natural hormone produced by the adrenal medulla, while the other enantiomer, the (S)-(+) isomer, has little or no biological activity (Figure 4.4). (The meaning and use of the (R) and (S) notation is described later in this chapter.)

Occasionally, the specific rotation of a compound can change over time. This phenomenon called *mutarotation* and is caused by a change in the molecular structure of the chiral compound. A good example of this can be seen with the monosaccharide glucose. α-D-(+)-glucose has an $[\alpha]$ value of +110°, while β-D-(+)-glucose has an $[\alpha]$ value of +19.7°. If freshly prepared solutions of α-D-(+)-glucose and β-D-(+)-glucose are allowed to stand, however, the $[\alpha]$ value of each compound slowly changes until an $[\alpha]$ value of +52.5° is reached. This is the $[\alpha]$ value for the equilibrium mixture of the two anomeric forms (which differ in configuration at carbon-1) of glucose. Both the α and the β pyranose forms of D-glucose are in equilibrium with a common open-chain form and this allows interconversion between the two cyclic forms. The equilibrium mixture obtained due to mutarotation of D-glucose has the approximate composition 33% α, 66% β and 1% open-chain aldehyde (Figure 4.5).

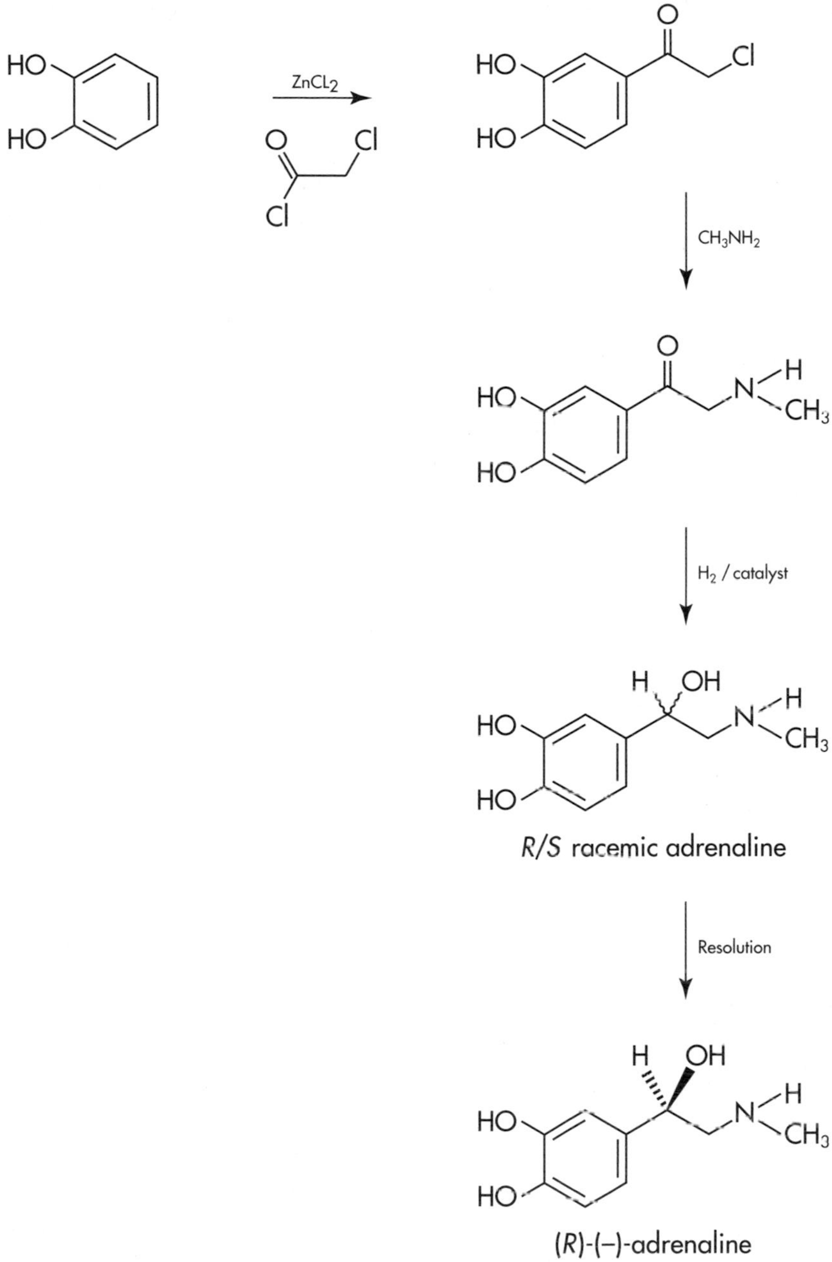

Figure 4.4 A synthesis of adrenaline (epinephrine).

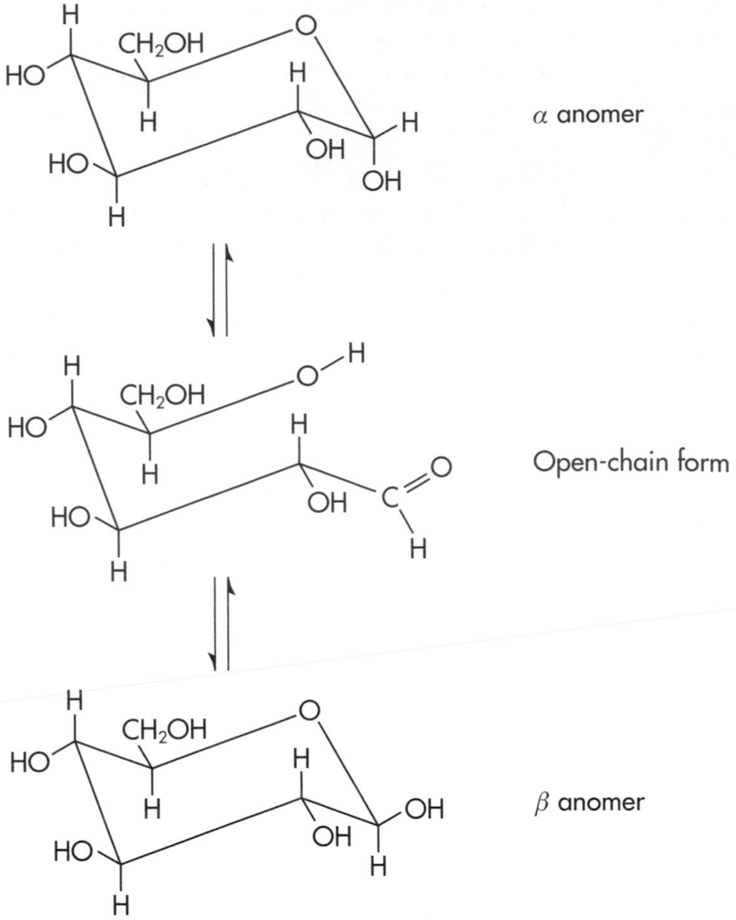

Figure 4.5 Mutarotation of D-glucose.

Biological systems

It is very important to realise that when drugs or medicines are administered to the body there is the opportunity for chiral interactions. This is because the human body is composed of enzymes and receptors that are protein in nature. These proteins are polymers of 20 or so naturally occurring amino acids. With the exception of glycine, all of these amino acids are chiral (all are L-series amino acids – see later) and it must be expected that a chiral drug will interact with these chiral receptors differently from its enantiomer. It is often the case that if a racemic mixture of a chiral drug is administered, only one enantiomer will be active, while the other will be less active or inactive, or may even be toxic. There is a school of thought among analysts that if a racemate is administered, and only one enantiomer is active at the receptor, then the patient has paid for and received 50% impurity and a clever lawyer may be able to pursue a claim!

A simple, non-invasive example of chiral discrimination can be seen using the smell of volatile compounds. (−)-Carvone is a natural product with the smell of spearmint oil. (+)-Carvone, the enantiomer, has the odour of caraway seeds (Figure 4.6). The fact that our noses can detect a different smell for the tiny concentration of each enantiomer present proves that our sense of smell is stereospecific. This is an example of a general rule, which is that the body is chiral and body systems can discriminate between enantiomers of chiral drugs. The history of drug development is littered with examples where the implications of stereochemistry were ignored (perhaps most tragically with the sedative thalidomide). Students of pharmacy and chemistry must expect the enantiomers of chiral drugs to interact differently with chiral receptors and enzymes.

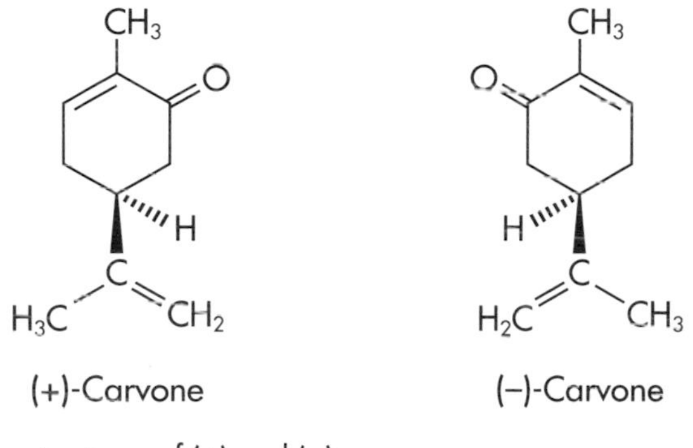

(+)-Carvone   (−)-Carvone

Figure 4.6   The structures of (+)-and (−)-carvone.

Fischer projections

It is sometimes useful to be able to draw a schematic diagram of the stereochemistry around a chiral carbon, especially when a molecule contains more than one chiral centre. The German chemist Emil Fischer solved this problem and his method of representing chiral centres is now called a Fischer projection.

A Fischer projection looks like a cross, with the chiral centre at the point where the lines cross. The horizontal lines are considered to be bonds projecting *towards* the viewer, while the two vertical lines are considered to project *away* from the viewer. In this way the tetrahedral arrangement of groups around an sp^3 hybridised carbon, for example, may be represented on a page in two dimensions. The other rule to remember when drawing a Fischer projection is to draw the carbon chain of the compound vertically *with the most oxidised carbon atom at the top*. An example of a Fischer projection of lactic acid, the acid produced when milk turns sour, is shown in Figure 4.7.

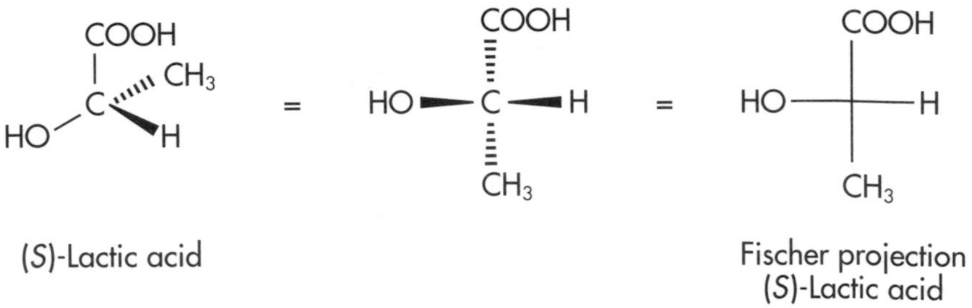

(S)-Lactic acid   Fischer projection
                                                                          (S)-Lactic acid

Figure 4.7   Fischer projection of lactic acid.

D and L configurations

The Fischer projection allows the stereochemistry around a chiral centre to be conveniently and accurately represented in two dimensions. Using the Fischer projection, a different system of describing the configuration (i.e. the arrangement in space of the atoms or groups attached to a chiral carbon) of groups around a chiral centre can now be introduced, the D and L convention. This method of describing absolute configuration is widely used in biochemistry and organic chemistry, particularly for carbohydrates and amino acids.

The simplest aldehyde-containing sugar (or aldose) is glyceraldehyde and this compound was selected as the standard compound for assigning the configuration of all carbohydrates. The dextrorotatory isomer of glyceraldehyde, (+)-glyceraldehyde, was arbitrarily assigned the absolute configuration shown in Figure 4.8. This was a lucky guess on the part of the chemists making the choice. They could not know at the time, with the analytical techniques at their disposal, how the atoms of glyceraldehyde were arranged in space around the chiral centre. Much later, when the technique of X-ray diffraction became available, it was possible to check the orientation of atoms in space in glyceraldehyde and it was found that the original guess had been correct.

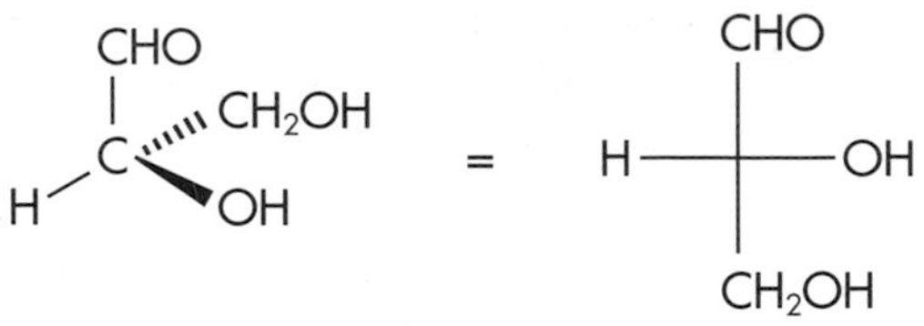

D-(+)-Glyceraldehyde

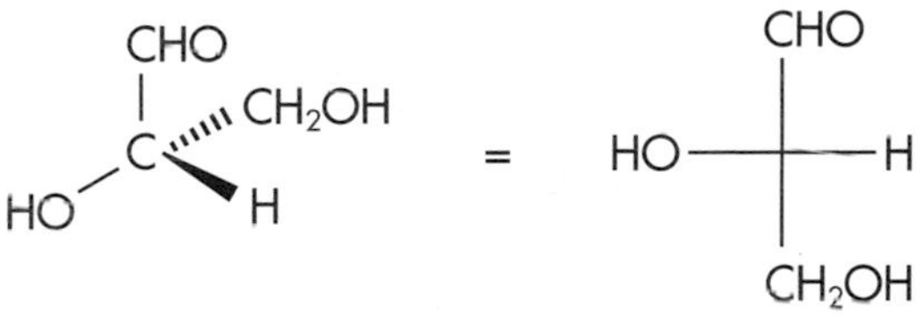

L-(−)-Glyceraldehyde

Figure 4.8   D and L forms of glyceraldehyde.

The Fischer projection of D-(+)-glyceraldehyde is shown in Figure 4.8. The carbon chain is drawn vertically, with the most oxidised carbon (the aldehyde) at the top. The OH group on the chiral centre is drawn on the *right-hand side* for the D isomer and on the *left-hand side* for the L isomer. It follows that any sugar that has the same stereochemistry as D-glyceraldehyde belongs to the D-series of sugars (e.g. D-glucose, D-galactose), while any sugar that has the same stereochemistry as L-glyceraldehyde belongs to the L-series of sugars.

For amino acids the situation is analogous. When the Fischer projection is drawn (carbon chain vertical with most oxidised carbon at the top) all of the 'natural' amino acids found in human proteins are found to have the NH_3^+ group on the left-hand side of the Fischer projection and therefore similar in configuration to L-(−)-glyceraldehyde. These amino acids are consequently known as L-series amino acids (Figure 4.9).

Amino acids of the opposite, D, configuration are known and do occur naturally in microorganisms. Indeed, the mode of action of penicillin antibiotics depends on the opposite stereochemistry of bacterial amino acids. In penicillin-sensitive bacteria, the organism manufactures a cell wall to contain the high osmotic pressure produced inside the bacterial cell. The bacterial cell wall consists of a polysaccharide (called *peptidoglycan*), which is reinforced by structural cross-linking of chains

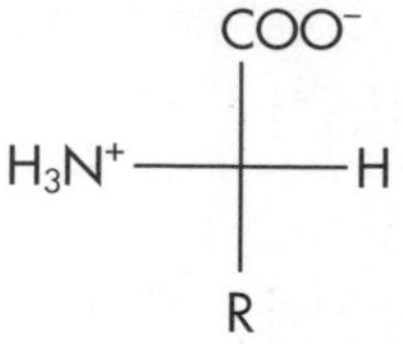

$$\begin{array}{c} COO^- \\ | \\ H_3N^+ \!\!\!-\!\!\!-\!\!\!-\!\!\!-\!\!\!-\!\! H \\ | \\ R \end{array}$$

Figure 4.9 Fischer projection of L-series amino acids.

of polypeptide. The situation is fairly complex, but the final step of the cross-linking is achieved by attaching the terminal amino acid of the cell wall, a glycine, to a D-alanine residue on an adjacent peptide chain. This cross-linking is catalysed by an enzyme called *transpeptidase* (or transaminase). Penicillins can inhibit the enzyme transpeptidase and prevent the formation of structural cross-links in the bacterial cell wall. The cell is weakened, becomes unable to contain the high internal osmotic pressure and bursts. Penicillin is able to inhibit the enzyme because of the close structural similarity between the penicillin anti-biotic and the D-alanine-D-alanine dipeptide from the cell wall. Penicillins are non-toxic to humans because we possess L-alanine, the amino acid with the opposite stereochemistry, in our proteins.

This is an example of an important concept in drug design called *selective toxicity*, which arises when a drug is poisonous to one type of organism (a bacterium in this case) but harmless to another (humans). Penicillins are a good example of selectively toxic drugs and, assuming the patient is not allergic to them, they are remarkably free of toxic side-effects. If a patient is allergic to penicillins, the macrolide antibiotic ery-thromycin is usually prescribed instead. The structures of penicillin and the D-alanine-D-alanine dipeptide are shown in Figure 4.10.

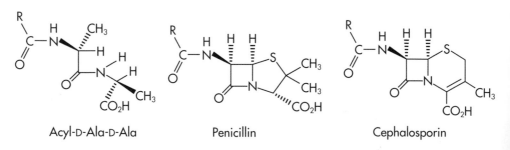

Acyl-D-Ala-D-Ala   Penicillin   Cephalosporin

Figure 4.10 The structures of D-alanine-D-alanine dipeptide, penicillin and cephalosporin.

Penicillins and the structurally similar class of antibiotic, the cephalosporins, are known collectively as *β-lactam antibiotics*. The β-lactam ring is the 4-membered cyclic amide ring common to both classes of antibiotics and fundamental to the molecular mode of action of the drugs. The β-lactam ring is under immense strain and opens easily if attacked by a nucleophile. This is because amides contain sp^2 hybridised carbon atoms, which normally have a bond angle of 120°. The bond angle of the amide in a β-lactam ring approaches 90°. A serine residue present in the active site of transpeptidase can attack the β-lactam ring, using the lone pair of electrons on the —OH, open the ring and so acylate the active site of the enzyme and prevent cell wall cross-linking (Figure 4.11).

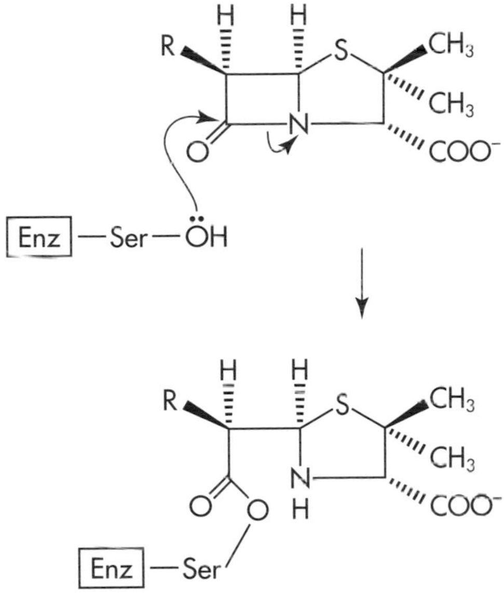

Figure 4.11   Mode of action of β-lactam antibiotics.

R and S configurations

The absolute configuration of atoms around a chiral centre may be drawn accurately by use of a Fischer projection and may be described (particularly in biochemistry for chiral carbohydrates and amino acids) by the D/L convention. The most successful system for displaying configuration of general compounds, however, is the Cahn–Ingold–Prelog convention, named for the three chemists who first described it. This system assigns each chiral centre in a molecule a letter (*R* or *S*) and is the method of choice when assigning the configuration of chiral centres of drug molecules.

To use the Cahn–Ingold–Prelog convention, a 'priority' is assigned to each group attached to the chiral centre according to the *atomic number* of the atom in question (NB not atomic weight – a common mistake). The numbering follows the atomic numbers in the periodic table, with heavy isotopes of the same atom taking priority over lighter ones. Hydrogen comes last, for example.

$$I > S > O > N > {}^{13}C > {}^{12}C > Li > {}^{3}H > {}^{2}H > {}^{1}H$$

If two groups cannot be distinguished on the basis of atomic number, the next atom of the group attached to the chiral centre is considered, and so on until the priorities are clear.

If a double- or triple-bonded group appears in the sequence, then each double bond is counted twice and each triple bond is counted three times, for example.

Once all the priorities around the chiral centre have been assigned, the molecule is viewed from the side *opposite the group with lowest priority* (usually hydrogen). If the order of the group priorities is arranged *clockwise* around the chiral centre, the chiral carbon receives the (R) configuration (from the Latin *rectus*). If the priority of groups is *anticlockwise* when viewed from the side opposite the group with lowest priority, the chiral centre is assigned (S) (from the Latin *sinister*, meaning 'to the left' – something to think about, all you readers who are left-handed!).

Students often find stereochemistry and the assigning of absolute configuration around a chiral centre difficult. This is usually because of difficulties picturing the arrangement of groups in space. The use of molecular models can be beneficial and they are recommended, particularly for beginners.

A number of worked tutorial examples and problems can be found on p. 96.

Molecules with more than one chiral centre

Since there are two possible configurations for an asymmetrically substituted carbon atom, a structure containing n such centres will, in theory, possess 2^n stereoisomers. The actual number of stereoisomers that exist may be less than this due to steric effects. Compounds that have the same stereochemistry at one chiral centre but different stereochemistry at the others are known as *diastereoisomers* (diastereomers); a good example is given by the alkaloids ephedrine and pseudoephedrine. Ephedrine (the (1*R*, 2*S*) diastereoisomer) is a natural product isolated from Ephedra (the *Ma Huang* plant) and known to Chinese medicine for over 3000 years. It was used last century for the treatment of asthma. Pseudoephedrine (the (1*S*, 2*S*) diastereoisomer) is a decongestant and a constituent of several 'over-the-counter' cold and flu remedies (Figure 4.12).

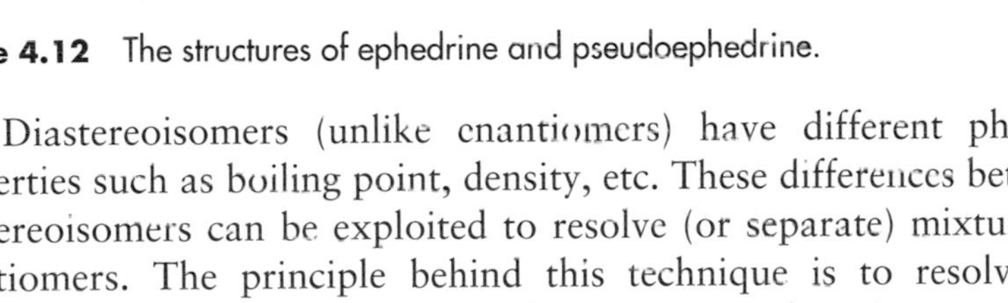

Figure 4.12 The structures of ephedrine and pseudoephedrine.

Diastereoisomers (unlike enantiomers) have different physical properties such as boiling point, density, etc. These differences between diastereoisomers can be exploited to resolve (or separate) mixtures of enantiomers. The principle behind this technique is to resolve the mixture of enantiomers by chemically converting them into a pair of diastereoisomers. This is achieved by reacting the racemic mixture with an optically pure reagent. These reagents are usually natural products; for example, if the racemic mixture contains acidic compounds, reaction is with an optically pure alkaloid such as strychnine or brucine.

Similarly, if the racemic mixture is composed of basic drugs, use is made of camphor-10-sulfonic acid, a natural product obtainable as an optically pure enantiomer. An example of the type of reactions involved is shown in Figure 4.13, where a pair of enantiomeric alcohols are resolved by reaction with phthalic anhydride and an optically pure base to form a pair of diastereoisomeric salts. Reactions of this type can be tedious to perform, and with the advent of HPLC with chiral stationary phases, are gradually being replaced.

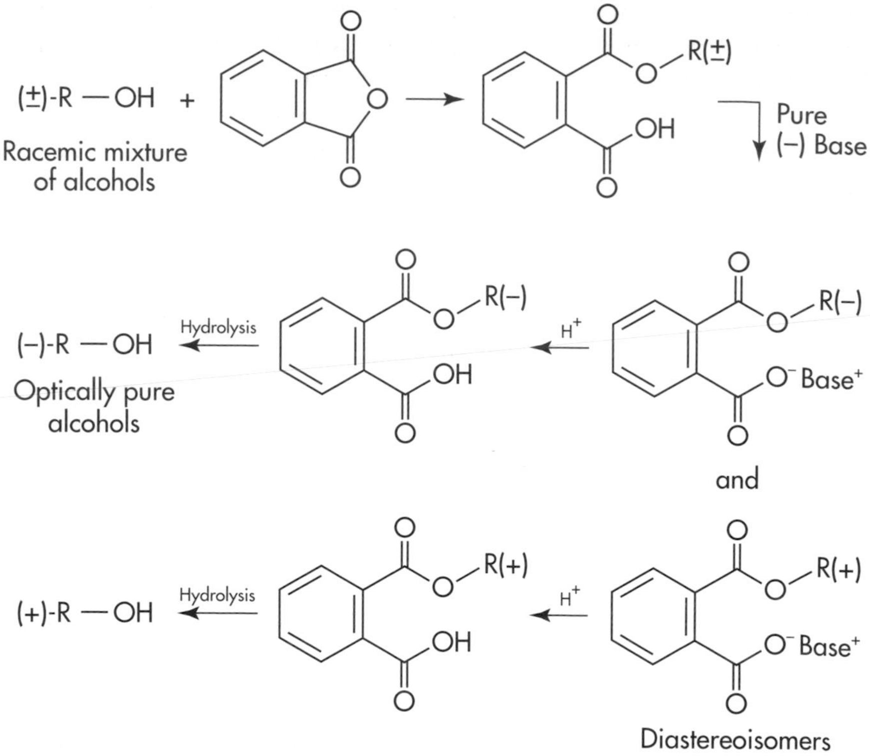

Figure 4.13 Resolution of a racemic mixture of alcohols.

Stereochemistry case study: thalidomide

The thalidomide disaster was the most serious drug-induced medical accident of the last 50 years. The drug was first marketed in Germany as a sedative with apparently few side-effects. It was considered safe and was indicated for the treatment of morning sickness associated with pregnancy. The drug was very popular and thousands of women around the world took thalidomide during their pregnancies. In the late 1950s and early 1960s a number of children were born with a serious congenital abnormality called *phocomelia*, characterised by deformities in limb structure or, in some cases, a total absence of a limb. Initially it was impossible to say what had caused the birth deformity, but eventually it was realised that all of the mothers involved had taken thalidomide at some time during their pregnancy. Official estimates put the number of children affected by thalidomide at 12 000, but this figure does not include the women who miscarried as a result of drug-induced damage to the fetus, so the true total is probably much higher.

Thalidomide caused birth deformities when tested (retrospectively) in rabbits and in primates, as well as humans, but tragically, the initial toxicology screen for the drug had been carried out in rats. It is now known that rats metabolise the drug differently from humans and, as a result, birth defects were not detected in the animal testing.

The structure of thalidomide is shown in Figure 4.14 with the chiral centre indicated.

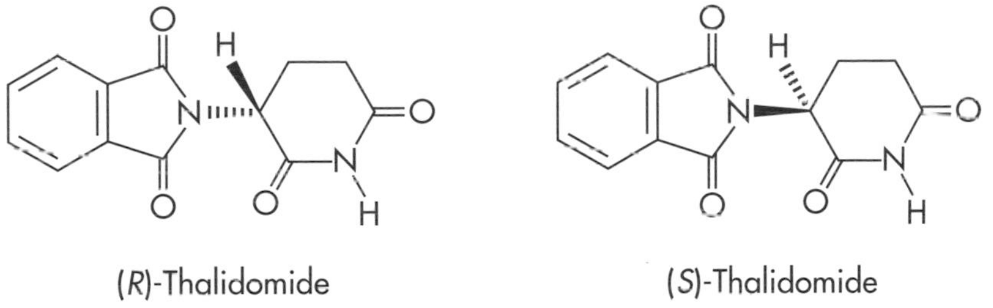

(R)-Thalidomide   (S)-Thalidomide

Figure 4.14   The enantiomers of thalidomide.

The drug was administered as the racemic mixture but, whereas the (R) isomer was an effective sedative, the opposite (S) isomer was found to have teratogenic properties and to cause deformities in the developing fetus. The toxic effect of thalidomide is most profound on new blood vessels developing in the fetus, a process called *angiogenesis*. The drug damages these delicate structures, transport of essential nutrients to the growing limbs is prevented and the limbs do not develop properly. The period of pregnancy when the symptoms of morning sickness are most severe coincides almost exactly with the period of most rapid limb growth in the fetus, so, unfortunately, the drug was taken at the worst possible time during the pregnancy to damage the fetus.

In cases of drug toxicity like this when one enantiomer is active (often called the *eutomer*)and the opposite enantiomer is toxic (called the *distomer*), the obvious solution is to resolve the racemic mixture into the two enantiomers and administer only the safe (R) isomer as a pure enantiomer. Unfortunately, it is now known that, in the case of thalidomide, administration of the enantiomerically pure (R) isomer would not have prevented the disaster since this isomer undergoes racemisation *in vivo*; in other words, administration of the pure enantiomer results in formation of a 50/50 racemic mixture in the bloodstream. The half-life for this reaction has been determined as 566 minutes at 37 °C and pH 7.4. This means that even if pure (R) isomer had been given, in a little less than ten hours half of it would have been converted into the toxic enantiomer. The situation is (even) more complicated because thalidomide is metabolised in the body and the metabolites themselves may be toxic.

The drug was withdrawn from the market as soon as evidence of the birth defects became known and for many years thalidomide disappeared from the Pharmacopoeia. Recently, however, thalidomide has undergone something of a renaissance and is now the drug of choice for erythema nodosum leprosum, a very severe inflammatory condition associated with leprosy. The drug is used only in male patients or in female patients who are not of child-bearing age.

Thalidomide is also undergoing trials as an adjuvant to cancer treatment, where the inhibition of angiogenesis may be employed to damage a tumour's blood supply and, hence, starve the tumour of oxygen and nutrients. There are also reports that the drug may possess immunomodulatory activity and may be of benefit in the treatment of autoimmune diseases such as Crohn's disease. It will be interesting to see whether thalidomide, after all the damage and misery it has caused, can become a useful and beneficial drug in the future.

Geometrical isomerism

Compounds that possess a multiple bond do not rotate easily about the bond. This gives rise to a type of isomerism called *geometrical* (or *cis–trans*) isomerism. If the substituents around the double bond are similar and both are on the same side of the double bond, the term *cis* is used to describe the molecule. If the same groups are on opposite sides of the double bond, the term *trans* is used to describe the configuration, as illustrated in Figure 4.15.

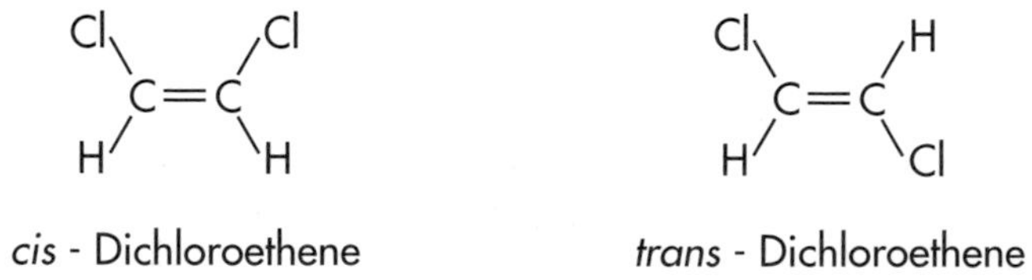

cis - Dichloroethene   *trans* - Dichloroethene

Figure 4.15 Examples of *cis* and *trans* isomerism.

The *cis–trans* convention is perfectly adequate for the description of simple compounds; however, for more complex examples a system based on the Cahn–Ingold–Prelog rules has been developed. The groups surrounding the double bond are assigned a Cahn–Ingold–Prelog priority depending on the atomic numbers of the substituents. The configuration in which the high-priority substituents are on the same side of the double bond is called the (*Z*) isomer (from the German *zusammen* meaning together). The alternative configuration, with the high-priority groups on opposite sides of the double bond, is described as (*E*) (also from the German. *entgegen* or opposite). Examples of (*Z*) and (*E*) isomers are shown in Figure 4.16.

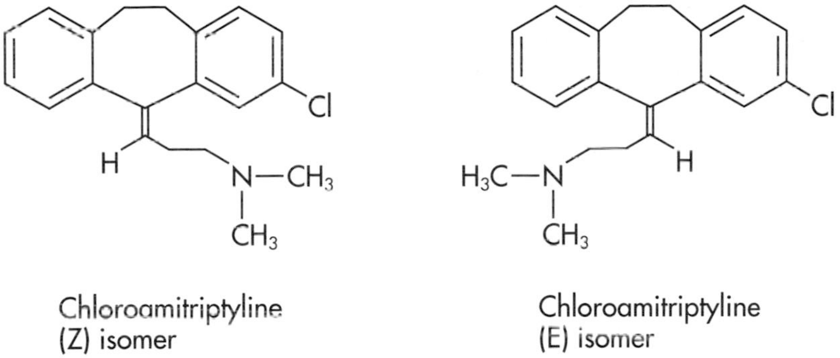
Cl
H
N—CH3
CH3
Chloroamitriptyline
(Z) isomer
Cl
H3C—N
H
CH3
Chloroamitriptyline
(E) isomer

Figure 4.16 Examples of (*Z*) and (*E*) isomers.

It should be obvious that the *cis* isomer is *usually* also the (*Z*) isomer, while the *trans* isomer is *usually* also the (*E*) isomer. This useful arrangement is not foolproof, however, and the anticancer drug tamoxifen is a notable example of a drug that is *trans* with respect to the phenyl groups, but also (*Z*) when the Cahn–Ingold–Prelog priorities are used (Figure 4.17).

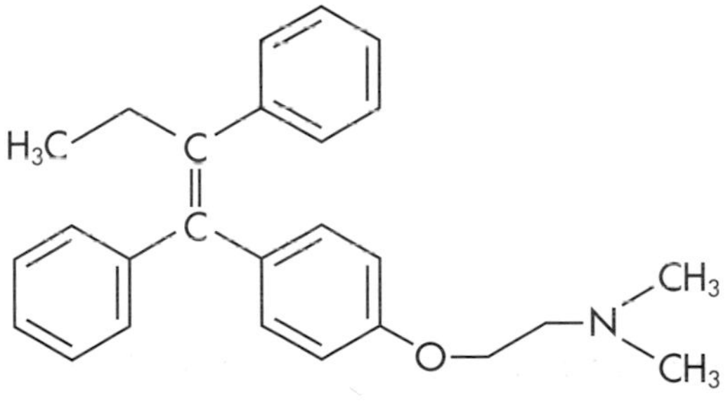
H3C
C
C
CH3
N
O
CH3

Figure 4.17 The structure of tamoxifen.

Tutorial examples

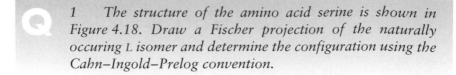

> **1** The structure of the amino acid serine is shown in Figure 4.18. Draw a Fischer projection of the naturally occuring L isomer and determine the configuration using the Cahn–Ingold–Prelog convention.

$$HOCH_2CH(\overset{+}{N}H_3)COO^-$$

Figure 4.18 The structure of serine.

A 1 A Fischer projection of serine is shown in Figure 4.19. The carbon chain is drawn vertical with the most oxidised carbon at the top. For the amino acid to be a member of the L-series the NH_3^+ group must be on the *left* of the Fischer projection. The priorities for the Cahn–Ingold–Prelog convention are also shown in Figure 4.19.

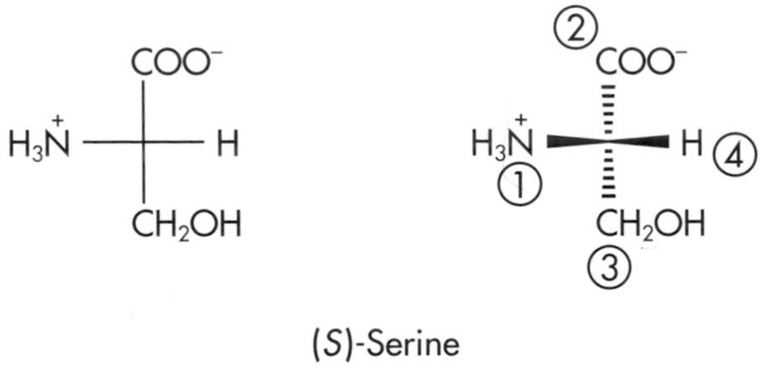

(*S*)-Serine

Figure 4.19 Fischer projection and Cahn–Ingold–Prelog convention for serine.

The highest priority is the NH_3^+, since the atomic number of nitrogen is 7; the second priority is COO^-; the third priority is the side-chain of the amino acid $-CH_2OH$; and the lowest priority (as always) is the hydrogen. The direction of rotation is therefore clockwise when viewed in the Fischer projection, but the Cahn–Ingold–Prelog convention demands that the chiral centre is viewed from the side *opposite* the group of lowest priority; therefore this molecule is (*S*). In fact, *all the common* L-*series amino acids are* (S) *unless the side-chain contains a sulfur atom.* This is because the group with the second priority is always the COO⁻ group unless there is an atom of higher atomic number than oxygen in the side-chain. In the case of the amino acid L-cysteine, the Cahn–Ingold–Prelog convention is (R) since one sulfur atom in the side-chain takes priority over the two oxygens in the COO⁻ group.

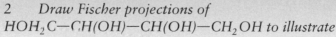

Q   2   *Draw Fischer projections of*
HOH₂C—CH(OH)—CH(OH)—CH₂OH to illustrate
(a)   A pair of enantiomers
(b)   A pair of diastereoisomers
(c)   A meso compound

A   2   The answers are shown in Figure 4.20. Structures (1) and (2) are enantiomeric pairs. Structures (1) and (3) and structures (2) and (3) are pairs of diastereoisomers (or diastereomers), while structure (c) is a meso compound. A meso compound is optically inactive since it possesses a plane of symmetry and is superimposable on its mirror image. It does, however, contain two chiral carbon atoms. This reminds us that *not all compounds that contain chiral centres are optically active.*

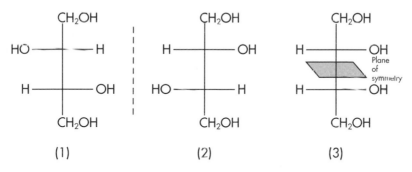

Figure 4.20 Enantiomers, diastereoisomers and a meso compound.

Problems

Q4.1   Four representations of the antidote dimercaprol, used in the treatment of heavy-metal poisoning, are shown in Figure 4.21. Assign each as either (R) or (S). Bonds projecting *out* of the page towards the reader are shown as solid wedges, while bonds projecting *into* the page are represented as dotted lines.

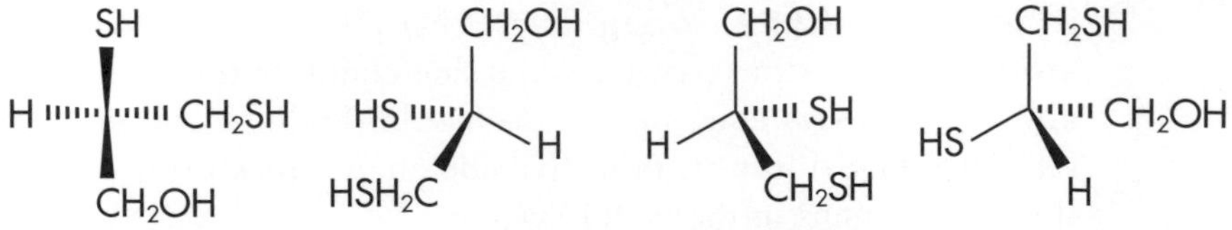

Figure 4.21 Representations of dimercaprol.

Q4.2 Designate each of the structures in Figure 4.22 as either (*E*) or (*Z*).

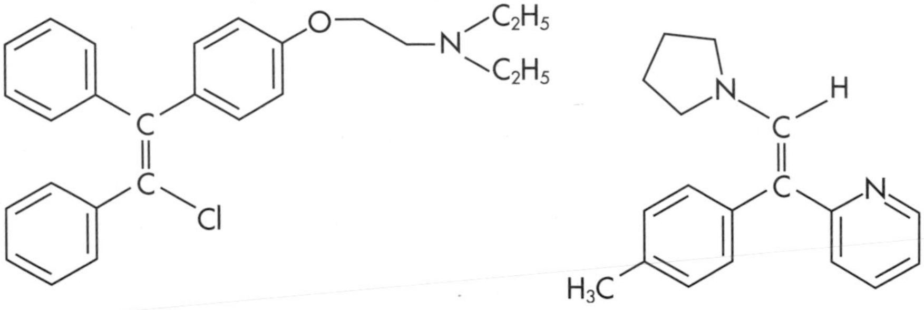

Figure 4.22 Structures of compounds that have geometrical isomers.

Q4.3 The structure of naloxone hydrochloride is shown in Figure 4.23. Assign the stereochemistry at the 5- and 14-positions using the Cahn–Ingold–Prelog convention.

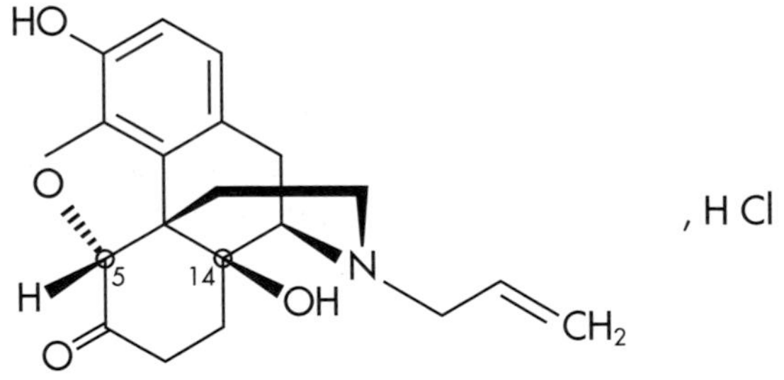

Figure 4.23 Structure of naloxone hydrochloride.

(Answers to problems can be found on pp. 219–220.)

5

Drug metabolism

When drugs and medicines are administered to a patient, it is rare for the drug molecule to emerge from the patient unchanged. Most of the foreign compounds (or *xenobiotics*) taken into the body undergo a variety of chemical changes brought about by enzymes in the liver, intestine, kidney, lung and other tissues. These transformations (especially oxidation reactions) may give rise to compounds (or *metabolites*) that are toxic. These metabolites are capable of reacting with important macromolecules within the body (such as DNA and proteins) to cause toxicity. An insight into the mechanisms that give rise to the formation of drug metabolites is therefore important from a drug safety point of view.

The body's main strategy for dealing with these xenobiotics is to convert the molecule into a more hydrophilic or water-soluble derivative, which can then be excreted via the kidneys in the urine. Reactions of this type are known collectively as *drug metabolism*, although the body systems that carry out these biotransformations arose through evolution long before drugs were taken therapeutically. Our ancestors were exposed throughout their lives to environmental poisons and foreign chemicals in their diet and mechanisms evolved to detoxify these agents and protect the body.

Today, the situation is, if anything, even more complex. Consumption of 'recreational' drugs such as tobacco and alcohol expose the body to thousands of foreign compounds, many of them potentially toxic. Environmental poisons such as pesticide residues in food and carcinogens (cancer-causing agents) produced by high-temperature cooking of fats and proteins in meat add to the cocktail of non-essential exogenous compounds absorbed by modern humans that may be harmful to their health. The consumption of drugs and medicines for therapeutic purposes must be viewed against this backdrop and a student must become familiar with the reactions involved in drug metabolism and the effects these biotransformations have on pharmacological activity, duration of action and toxicity of drugs.

Metabolic pathways

Foreign compounds such as drugs taken into the body undergo enzymatic transformations, which usually result in a loss of pharmacological activity. This is known as *detoxification*. Occasionally, the action of these enzymes may convert an inactive compound (or prodrug) into a pharmacologically active compound. In this case, the process is described as *bioactivation*. Prodrugs are pharmacologically inactive derivatives of the active molecule that are designed to break down within the body to release the active drug. The prodrug approach is often used in pharmacy to overcome problems such as poor absorption or instability when the parent drug is given orally, or if the parent drug has an unpalatable taste or smell that needs to be disguised.

There are two main types of biotransformation observed in the body, imaginatively called *Phase 1* and *Phase 2* reactions, although many drugs undergo both types of process.

Phase 1 reactions are reactions in which a new functional group is introduced into the molecule, or an existing group is converted into another (usually more water-soluble) derivative. Phase 2 reactions (conjugations) are where an existing functional group in the molecule is masked by the addition of a new group. The conjugate is formed between the drug and a hydrophilic compound such as glucuronic acid and the resulting conjugate (a glucuronide) will usually be much more water soluble than the parent drug. Most drugs are hydrophobic and so not inherently water soluble. Metabolism to a more water-soluble and less toxic derivative terminates drug action and allows the body to excrete the drug easily in the urine. If the administered drug is already hydrophilic, the molecule is often excreted unchanged.

The processes involved in drug metabolism involve simple chemical reactions such as oxidation (the most common), reduction and dealkylation and are influenced by a number of factors including:

- *Genetic factors.* Differences are observed between species (important since most medicines intended for human use are tested first in animals) and between individuals in a population.
- *Physiological factors.* These include age of the patient, gender, pregnancy and nutritional status. Very young patients whose livers have not developed fully and very old patients whose liver function has deteriorated metabolise drugs more slowly than the normal adult population. There are also differences in the rates of metabolism between men and women and between pregnant and non-pregnant women. The causes of these effects are unknown but are probably due to differences in levels of circulating sex hormones.

- *Pharmacodynamic factors.* These were mentioned briefly in Chapters 2 and 3 and include dose, frequency and route of administration and extent of protein binding.
- *Environmental factors.* Examples of these are co-administration of other drugs, which can effect the rate and extent of drug metabolism. This can become literally a matter of life and death as a number of potentially fatal drug interactions involve liver enzyme induction and competition for drug-metabolism enzymes.

Cytochromes P450

The most important and most extensively studied drug metabolism system in the body is the family of cytochrome P450 monooxygenases (CYP450). Many different forms of these enzymes exist (called *iso-forms*), although they are all membrane-bound mixed-function oxidases located on the smooth endoplasmic reticulum of the liver. CYP450 acts as a very sophisticated electron transport system responsible for the oxidative metabolism of a large number of drugs and other xenobiotics. It accomplishes this due to the presence of an ion of iron at the active site that can accept or donate electrons to allow oxidation reactions to take place. The iron in CYP450 can exist in a number of oxidation states, of which Fe^{2+} (ferrous) and Fe^{3+} (ferric) are the most important.

A detailed description of the (fascinating) molecular mode(s) of action of this important enzyme system is beyond the scope of this book and the interested reader should consult textbooks of biochemistry, pharmacology or medicinal chemistry for more information. What is important is that a student should understand the functional group interconversions brought about by CYP450 and appreciate the metabolic effects of these changes on the physicochemical properties of drugs.

The oxidations brought about by CYP450 may be simple oxidation of a part of the drug molecule, e.g. a side-chain or aromatic ring, or may involve more complicated transformations in which a functional group is lost from the molecule in the course of the oxidation reaction. Examples of this type of transformation are O- and N-dealkylations (in which an alkyl group is lost) and deaminations (in which an amino group is lost). Examples of the types of transformation catalysed by CYP450 are shown in Table 5.1. This list is not intended to be exhaustive, it merely indicates the range of chemical interconversions catalysed by this enzyme system.

Table 5.1 Oxidative biotransformations catalysed by CYP450

Substrate	*Product(s)*

1. Side-chain oxidation

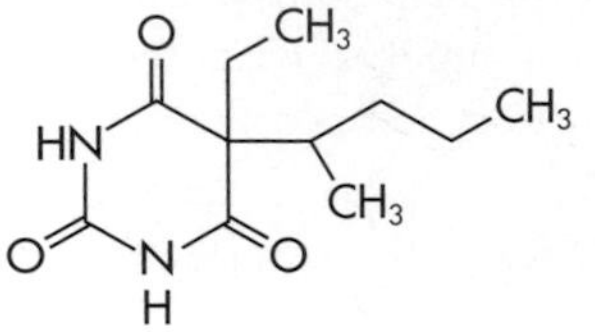

Pentobarbital

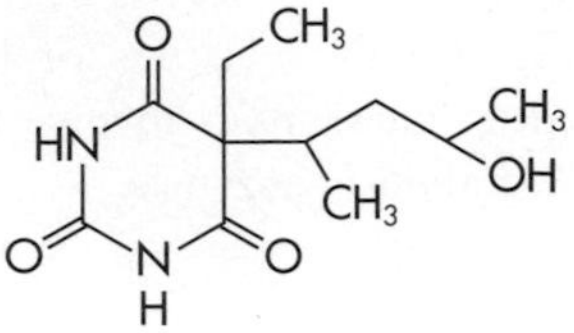

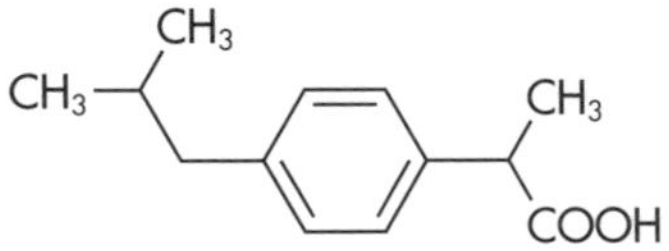

Ibuprofen

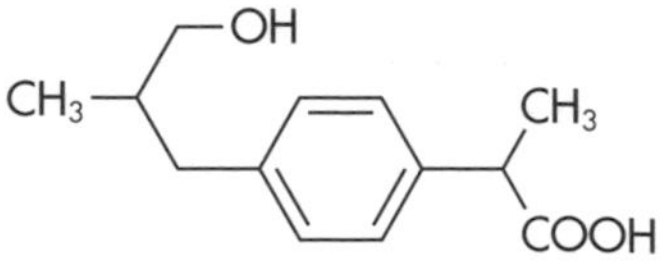

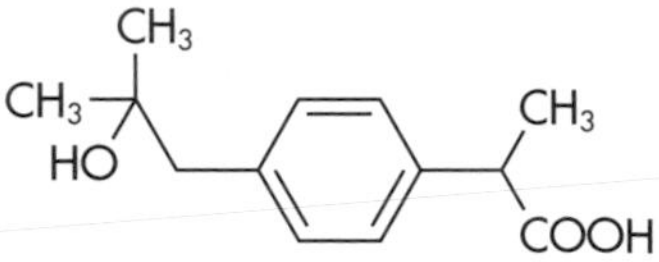

2. Aromatic ring oxidation

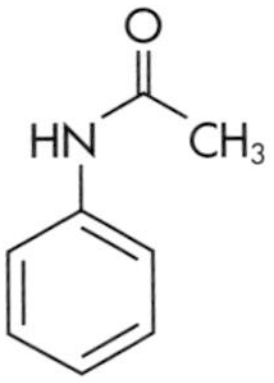

Acetanilide

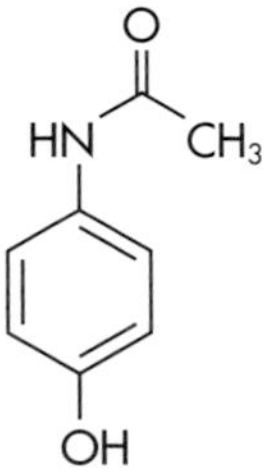

Paracetamol

3. Methyl oxidation

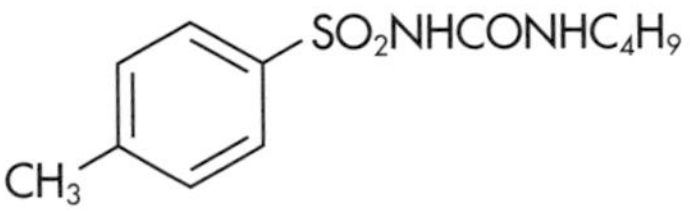

Tolbutamide

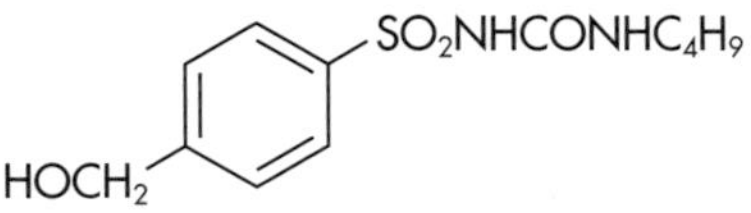

(*continued*)

Table 5.1 *Continued*

Substrate	*Product(s)*

4. Heterocyclic ring oxidation

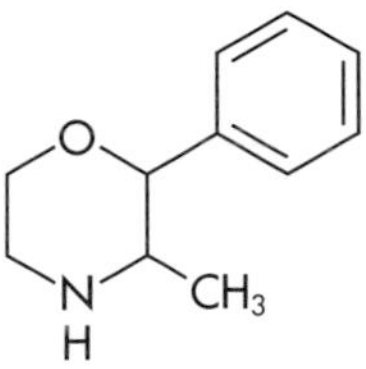

Phenmetrazine

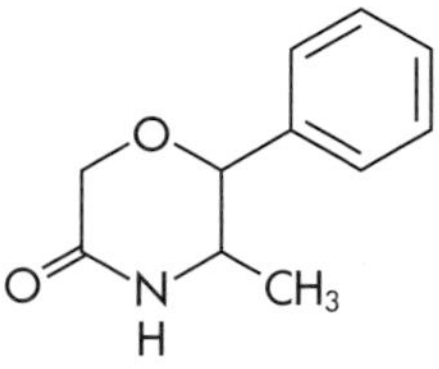

5. N-Dealkylation

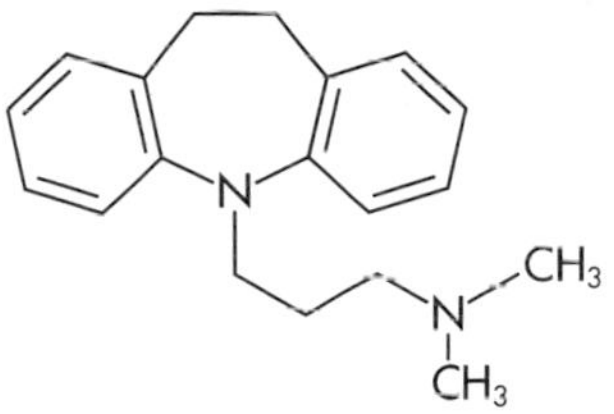

Imipramine

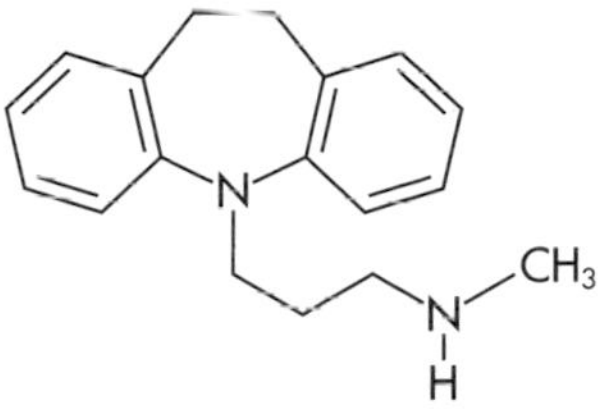

Desipramine

6. O-Dealkylation

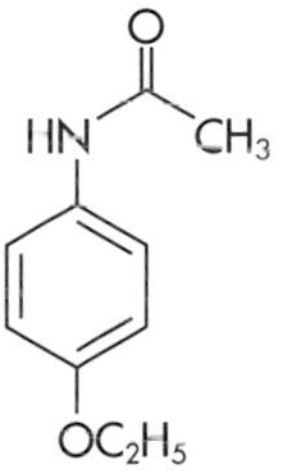

Phenacetin

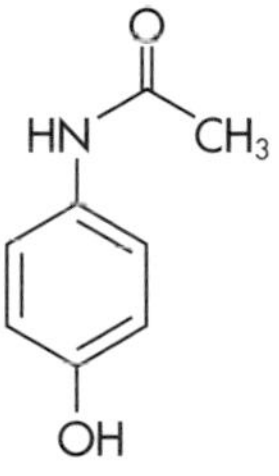

Paracetamol

7. S-Dealkylation

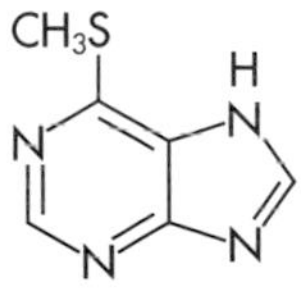

6-Methylmercaptopurine

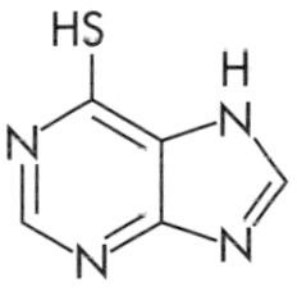

6-Mercaptopurine

(*continued*)

Table 5.1 *Continued*

Substrate	*Product(s)*

8. Deamination

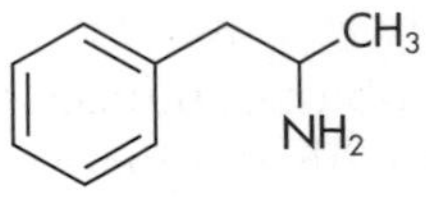

Amfetamine

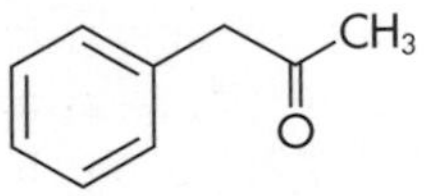

+ NH_4^+

9. N-Oxidation

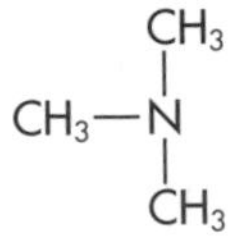

Trimethylamine

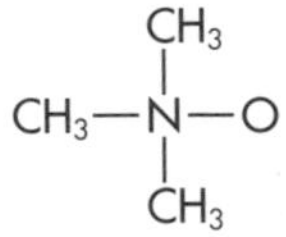

Trimethylamine oxide

10. Sulfoxidation

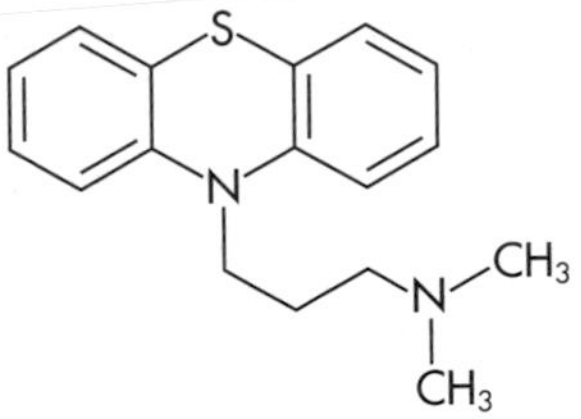

Chlorpromazine

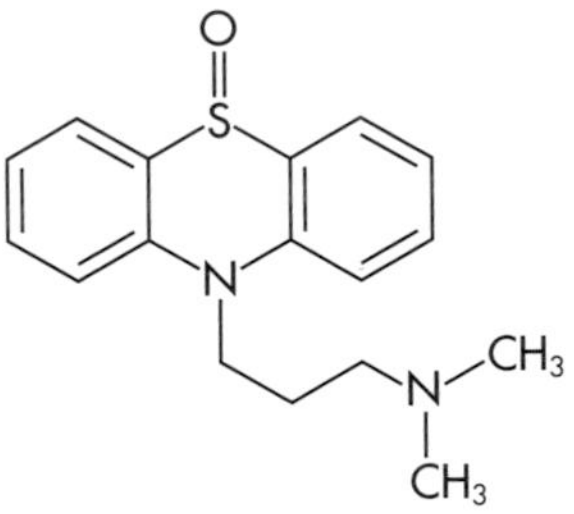

Chlorpromazine sulfoxide

11. Azoreduction

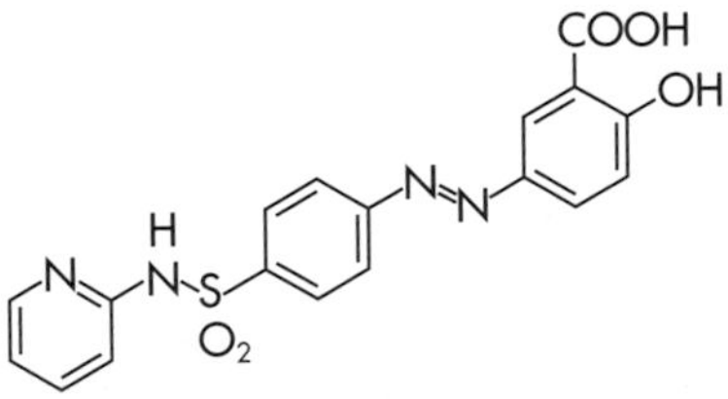

Sulfasalazine

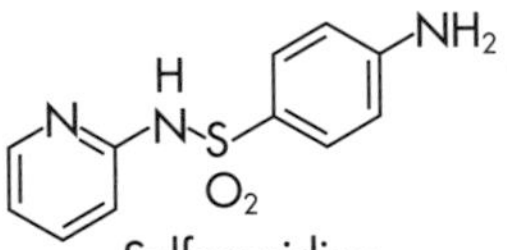

Sulfapyridine

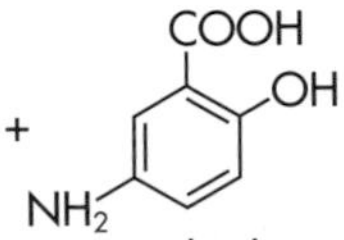

+

5-Aminosalicylic acid

Enzyme induction and inhibition

Many drugs and environmental compounds can enhance their own metabolism and that of other compounds. Prolonged administration of a xenobiotic can lead to an increased rate of metabolism of a wide variety of compounds. This process is known as *enzyme induction* and is dose-dependent. In effect, administration of a xenobiotic induces the synthesis of more enzyme by the organism to deal with the increased metabolic challenge caused by the xenobiotic. The increased levels of enzyme can metabolise not only the xenobiotic causing the induction but also other drugs metabolised by that enzyme system. The CYP450 enzyme system is responsible for a large number of biotransformations, so the possibility of drug interactions is very large.

Environmental chemicals such as polycyclic aromatic hydrocarbons (PAHs), present in cigarette smoke, xanthines and flavones in foods, halogenated hydrocarbons in insecticides and food additives can all alter the activity of CYP450 enzymes. Drugs that can cause CYP450 induction include antibiotics such as rifampicin and erythromycin, anticonvulsants such as phenobarbital and phenytoin and recreational drugs such as ethanol. Co-administration of enzyme inducers along with other drugs (particularly drugs with a narrow therapeutic index, e.g. warfarin) can result in increased rates of metabolism of the drug and, consequently, a reduction in duration of action and therapeutic effect.

Not only can drug-metabolising enzymes be induced by xenobiotics, they can also be inhibited. In this case, administration of xenobiotic results in decreased rate of metabolism of the xenobiotic and any co-administered drug. Drugs interacting in this way with CYP450 include the histamine H_2-receptor antagonist, cimetidine, the azole antifungals (ketoconazole, fluconazole, etc.) and the calcium channel blocker diltiazem. If drug metabolism is inhibited, the duration of action and plasma concentrations of co-administered drug will be increased, potentially leading to the appearance of side-effects and drug toxicity. CYP450 inhibitors can be split into three categories according to their mechanism of action.

- *Reversible inhibitors*, such as cimetidine, which interact with the complexed iron at the active site of the enzyme to inhibit oxidation of other drugs. The inhibition occurs before any oxidation of the inhibitor occurs and is reversible once the inhibitor is removed.
- *Metabolite intermediate complexation of CYP450.* In this the drug is acted upon by the enzyme to form an oxidised derivative with a high affinity for the iron at the active site. Examples of this type of inhibition include alkylamine drugs that undergo oxidation to nitrosoalkane derivatives. Inhibition of this

type renders the enzyme unavailable for further oxidation and synthesis of new enzyme is required to restore CYP450 activity.

- *Mechanism-based inactivation of CYP450 (or suicide inhibition)* occurs when a non-toxic drug is metabolised by CYP450 to generate a metabolite that can bind irreversibly with the enzyme. The mechanism of inhibition usually involves free-radical alkylation or acylation of the active site and results in destruction of enzyme activity. Examples of drugs that act in this way include the antibiotic chloramphenicol and the anticancer agent cyclophosphamide.

Drug conjugation reactions (Phase 2)

Conjugation reactions are very important in the biotransformation of drugs and foreign chemicals within the body. Conjugation reactions involve the attachment of very hydrophilic species such as glucuronic acid or glycine to xenobiotics and are usually considered to terminate pharmacological action. The drug conjugate is much less lipophilic and much more water soluble and is excreted easily by the kidneys. The situation is complicated, however, because drugs can be a substrate for more than one metabolising enzyme and there is no 'pecking order' or priority for enzyme action. This sequential conjugation can give rise to a bewildering array of metabolites and conjugates appearing in the urine or faeces when a drug is administered.

The major routes for drug conjugation are shown below.

Glucuronic acid conjugation

This is perhaps the most common route of Phase 2 drug metabolism because of the high levels of glucuronic acid in the liver and the relatively large number of functional groups that can act as a substrate for conjugate formation (alcohols, phenols, carboxylic acids, amines). The xenobiotic (or its Phase 1 metabolite) reacts with the activated form of glucuronic acid (uridine diphosphate glucuronic acid, or UDPGA) to give a derivative called a *glucuronide* as shown in Figure 5.1.

The glucuronide derivatives formed in this way are much more water soluble than the parent drug. This is due to the large number of polar OH groups and a carboxylate group that will ionise at neutral pH. The glucuronide derivatives are less active pharmacologically and more easily excreted than the drug itself. Glucuronic acid conjugation is therefore, for most drugs, an example of a process that terminates drug action. An important exception to this is the analgesic morphine. This important drug forms a 3-O- and a 6-O-glucuronide, both of which are active at opiate receptors in the body (see Figure 5.2). The overall

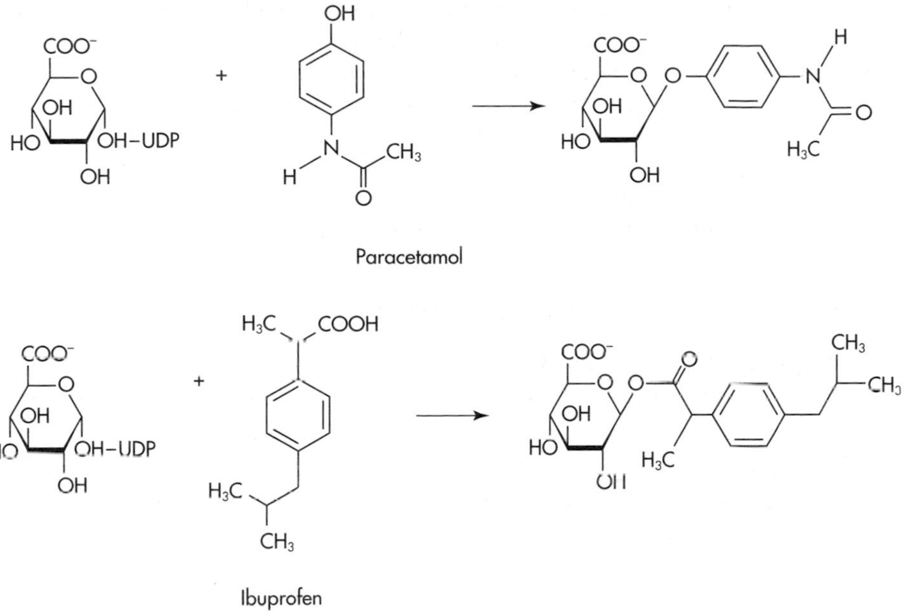

Figure 5.1   Formation of glucuronides.

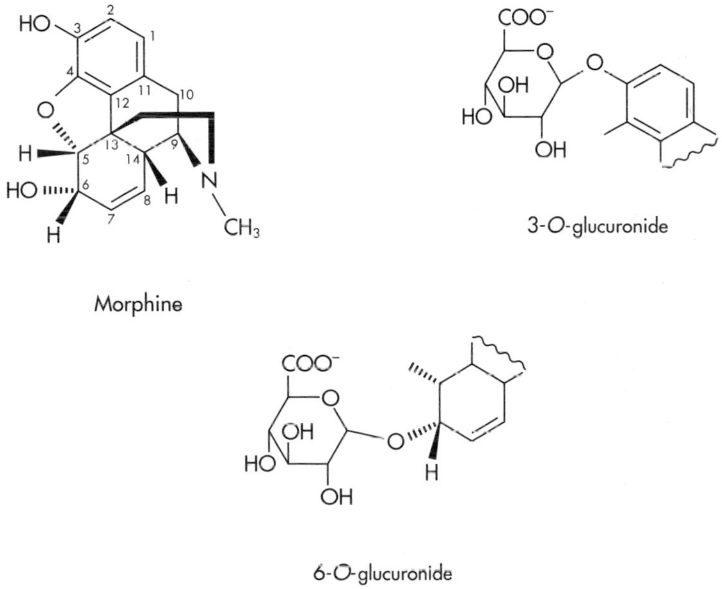

Figure 5.2   The structures of morphine and its 3-*O*- and 6-*O*-glucuronides.

analgesic effect of morphine is a combination of the action of the drug and the effects of both active glucuronides and is, as a result, very complex.

Sulfate conjugation

Drugs and hormones that contain the phenolic functional group are metabolised by conjugation to a sulfate group (a process called sulfation). Examples of compounds metabolised in this way include the neurotransmitter noradrenaline (norepinephrine) as well as hormones such as adrenaline (epinephrine), thyroxine and some steroids. In addition, the phenolic OH of tyrosine residues in proteins can act as a substrate for sulfation reactions, leading to a change in the physicochemical properties of the peptide or protein. The sulfur source is inorganic sulfate, which combines with ATP to form 3'-phosphoadenosine-5'-phosphosulfate (PAPS) and two phosphate groups. The enzyme sulfotransferase then attaches the sulfate group to the phenolic OH of the drug or hormone (Figure 5.3).

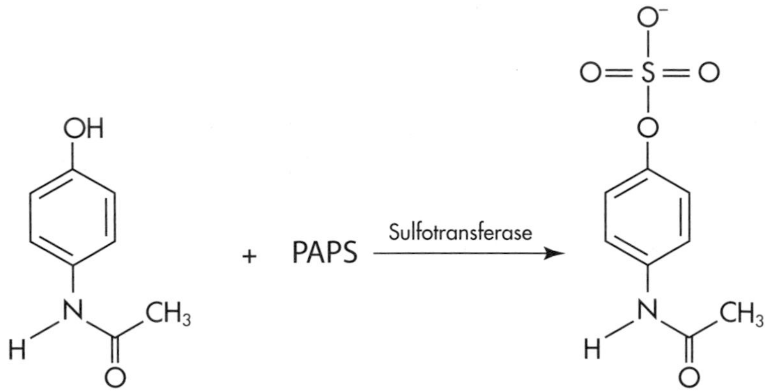

Figure 5.3   Sulfation of paracetamol.

If the dose of drug is high, the sulfate pathway can become saturated and other conjugation reactions (such as glucuronide formation) can take over. This is because the reservoir of inorganic sulfate in the body is finite and is easily overloaded.

The principal sites for sulfation reactions are the liver and kidneys, although an important site, especially after oral administration of drugs, is the small intestine. Sulfation in the gut can seriously affect the bioavailability of some drugs such as paracetamol (see Figure 5.3) and is the main reason why adrenaline (epinephrine) is not effective when given orally.

The sulfate conjugate of a drug is much more water soluble than the parent compound and is usually filtered by the kidneys and excreted in the urine. An important exception is steroid drugs, which are sulfated then excreted into the bile.

Amino acid conjugation

Conjugation with amino acids is an important route of Phase 2 metabolism for xenobiotics containing a carboxylic acid functional group. The amino acids involved include glycine (the simplest and most common α-amino acid), glutamine and taurine. Conjugation occurs with formation of a peptide bond between a carboxyl group of the drug and the NH_2 group of the amino acid after the xenobiotic has been activated by reaction with acetyl-coenzyme A. The major class of drug metabolised by this route is that of the non-steroidal anti-inflammatory drugs (NSAIDs) such as ibuprofen and ketoprofen. If the NSAID is chiral, conjugation with amino acid often results in inversion of the chiral centre. The reaction is illustrated in Figure 5.4 using benzoic acid as substrate. The product, hippuric acid, is present in human urine but was first isolated from the urine of horses and was named from the Greek word for horse, *hippos*. The amino acid conjugate of a drug is almost always more polar and more water-soluble than the parent molecule.

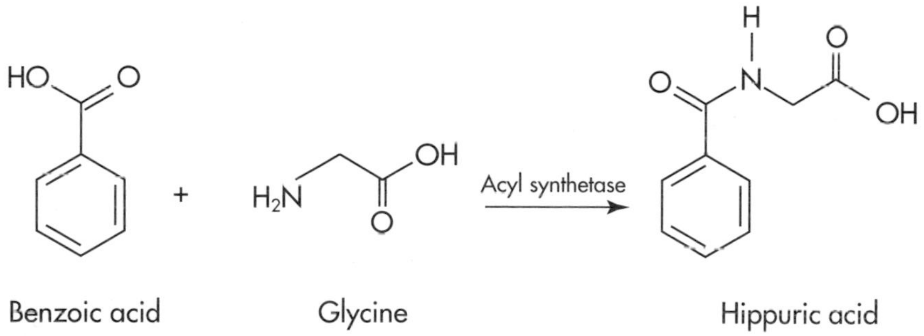

Figure 5.4   Glycine conjugation of benzoic acid.

Miscellaneous conjugation reactions

Several other types of conjugation reaction exist in the Phase 2 metabolism of drugs. Compounds possessing an amino group often undergo N-acetylation, primarily in the liver although other sites are known. The rate at which some patients carry out acetylations is known to vary, with the population dividing into *fast acetylators* who can form N-acetyl derivatives quickly and so terminate drug action, and *slow acetylators* who cannot perform the transformation so rapidly and accumulate the drug. These two subgroups of the population display differences in the rates of metabolism of a number of drugs including procainamide and isoniazid (shown in Figure 5.5). N-Acetylation of an amine is unusual in that the product formed is generally less water soluble than the parent amine, particularly if the solution is slightly acidic. This exception to the rule of 'metabolism to a more water-soluble derivative' can be rationalised as a termination of pharmacological action at the receptor. Acetylation of an amine removes a key hydrogen-bonding site (the nitrogen lone pair of electrons) from the drug and hence destroys one of the specific three-dimensional interactions with the target macromolecule.

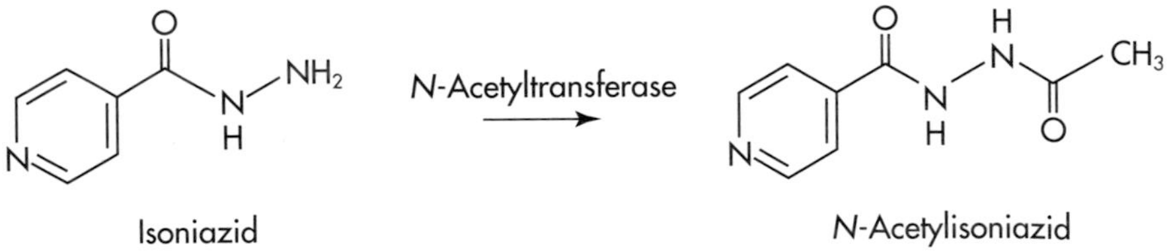

Figure 5.5   *N-Acetylation of isoniazid.*

Glutathione is another endogenous compound often found in drug conjugates. Glutathione is a tripeptide (γ-GluCysGly) found in high concentration in the liver. See Figure 5.6. The thiol group of glutathione is able to react with electrophilic drugs to protect other cell nucleophiles (such as DNA and proteins) from attack. This is often a detoxifying mechanism as in the case of N-acetylquinoneimine formed from paracetamol and epoxides formed as a result of CYP450 metabolism of double bonds (Figure 5.7).

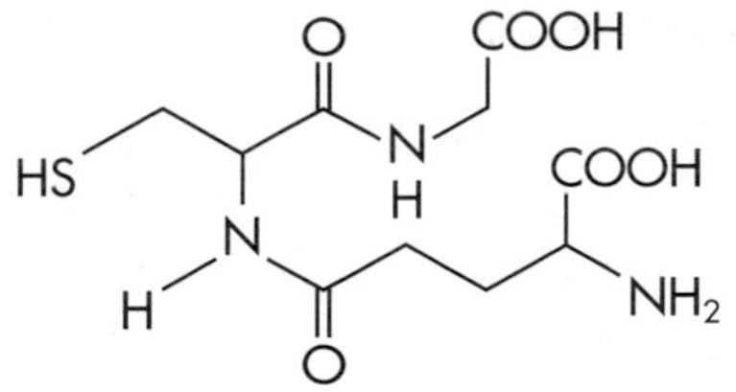

Figure 5.6   The structure of glutathione.

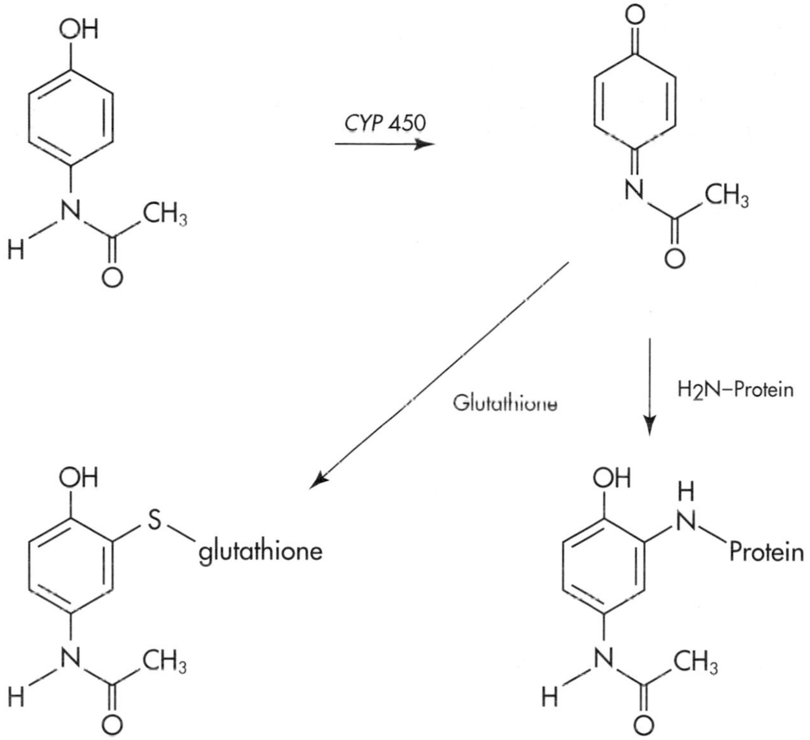

Figure 5.7   Role of glutathione in toxicity of paracetamol.

Paracetamol is the most popular 'over-the-counter' analgesic for adults and children on sale in the UK and is perfectly safe when taken at the recommended dosage (for an adult, currently not more that eight 500 mg tablets in any 24-hour period). When taken orally, paracetamol is quickly absorbed and transported in the bloodstream to the liver, where it is oxidised (by a CYP450 isoform) to *N*-acetyl-*p*-benzoquinoneimine as shown in Figure 5.7. This compound is reactive and will arylate essential cellular macromolecules (such as proteins), leading to toxicity that if untreated can cause liver failure and the need for transplantation. When paracetamol is taken at the approved dosage, there are sufficient levels of glutathione present in the body to reduce the toxic quinoneimine back to paracetamol. However, if paracetamol is taken in overdose, the levels of quinoneimine exceed the ability of glutathione to convert it back to paracetamol and toxicity to the liver results. In some cases, if treatment is not initiated in time, severe toxicity results, leading to death by acute liver failure. Treatment of paracetamol overdose is by administration of *N*-acetylcysteine (Figure 5.8). This compound (the acetyl derivative of the essential amino acid cysteine) functions as an alternative source of thiol (—SH) groups, which act in a similar manner to glutathione to detoxify the quinoneimine.

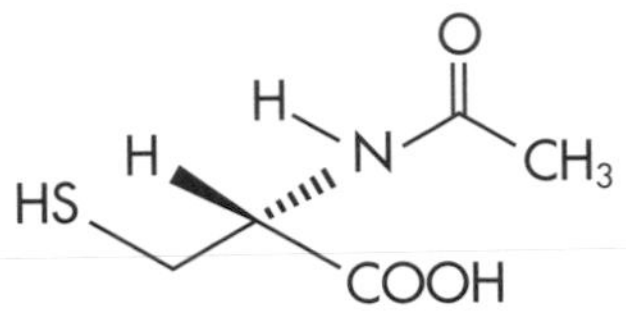

Figure 5.8 The structure of *N*-acetylcysteine.

A number of oxygen-, nitrogen- and sulfur- containing drugs can be metabolised by addition of a methyl group. O-Methylation and N-methylation are the most common reactions and are catalysed by methyltransferase enzymes such as catechol O-methyltransferase (COMT), one of the enzymes involved in terminating the action of adrenaline (epinephrine) and noradrenaline (norepinephrine). As in the case of acetylation reactions above, the O-methyl and N-methyl derivatives are more lipophilic and less water soluble than the parent drug. This metabolic transformation should also be viewed as a method of terminating pharmacological action rather than as a means of increasing water solubility prior to excretion by the kidneys. N-Methylation reactions are less common, although serotonin, histamine and tyramine are examples of endogenous hormones metabolised by methylation of the nitrogen.

Stereochemistry

Drug metabolism may be influenced by stereochemical factors if the molecule in question possesses one or more chiral centres. Examples of drugs that show stereochemical differences in rates of metabolism include α-methyldopa (where the (S) isomer is decarboxylated more rapidly than the (R) isomer) and the enantiomers of warfarin, which are reduced at different rates. The well-known endogenous compound mevalonic acid (3,5-dihydroxy-3-methylpentanoic acid) is chiral and exists as two enantiomers. When a racemic mixture of mevalonic acid is fed to animals, one optical isomer is absorbed and metabolised, while virtually all of the other isomer is excreted by the kidneys into the urine.

The fact that different rates of metabolism are observed when chiral drugs are used should not come as a surprise. Biotransformations are carried out in the body by enzymes, such as CYP450. These enzymes are themselves chiral since they are proteins and are composed of amino acids, which are, with the exception of glycine, all chiral. A chiral enzyme will, in general, interact differently with each enantiomer of a chiral drug. This effect is so widespread as to be considered normal. Almost all drug–macromolecule interactions occurring in the body show chiral discrimination. This is true whether they are drug–enzyme or drug–receptor in nature.

The situation is complicated further because some drugs show stereoselective absorption, distribution and excretion between enantiomers and it is difficult to determine which effects are due solely to metabolism and which are due to other biopharmaceutical factors.

Metabolic pathways for common drugs

Drug metabolism is a complex subject. The range of small molecules used in medicine is huge and the number and extent of biotransformations carried out by the body are vast. It is impossible in this book to detail each metabolite of every drug used therapeutically, but Table 5.2 lists some common drugs and their metabolic pathways. This table should not be memorised (!) but rather used as a means of illustrating the range and diversity of compounds used as drugs and the many transformations carried out within the body.

Table 5.2 Common metabolic pathways

Drug	Pathway
Amfetamines	Deamination (followed by oxidation and reduction of the ketone form
	N-oxidation
	N-dealkylation
	Hydroxylation of the aromatic ring
	Hydroxylation of the β-carbon atom
	Conjugation with glucuronic acid of the acid and alcohol products from ketone formed by deamination
Barbiturates	Oxidation and complete removal of substituents at carbon–5
	N-dealkylation at N^1 and N^3
	Desulfuration at carbon-2 (thiobarbiturates)
	Scission of the barbiturate ring at the 1:6 bond to give substituted malonylureas
Phenothiazines	N-dealkylation in the N^{10} side-chain
	N-oxidation in the N^{10} side-chain
	Oxidation of the heterocyclic S atom to sulfoxide or sulfone
	Hydroxylation of one or both aromatic rings
	Conjugation of phenolic metabolites with glucuronic acid or sulfate
	Scission of the N^{10} side-chain
Sulfonamides	Acetylation at the N^4 amino group
	Conjugation with glucuronic acid or sulfate at the N^4 amino group
	Acetylation or conjugation with glucuronic acid at the N^1 amino group
	Hydroxylation and conjugation in the heterocyclic ring, R
Phenytoin	Hydroxylation of one aromatic ring
	Conjugation of phenolic products with glucuronic acid or sulfate
	Hydrolytic scission of the hydantoin ring at the bond between carbons-3 and 4 to give 5,5-diphenylhydantoic acid

(*continued*)

Table 5.2 *Continued*

Drug	Pathway
Pethidine	Hydrolysis of ester to acid
	N-dealkylation
	Hydroxylation of aromatic ring
	N-oxidation
	Both N-dealkylation and hydrolysis
	Conjugation of phenolic products

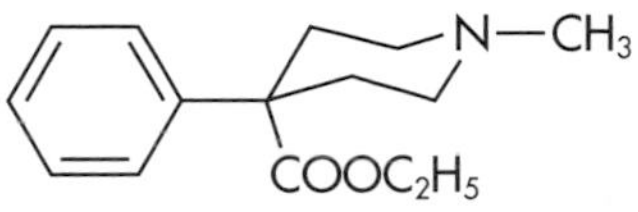

Pethidine structure with N—CH₃ and COOC₂H₅

	Pathway
Pentazocine	Hydroxylation of terminal methyl groups of the alkenyl side-chain to give *cis* and *trans* (major) alcohols
	Oxidation of hydroxymethyl product of the alkenyl side chain to carboxylic acids
	Reduction of alkenyl side-chain and oxidation of terminal methyl group

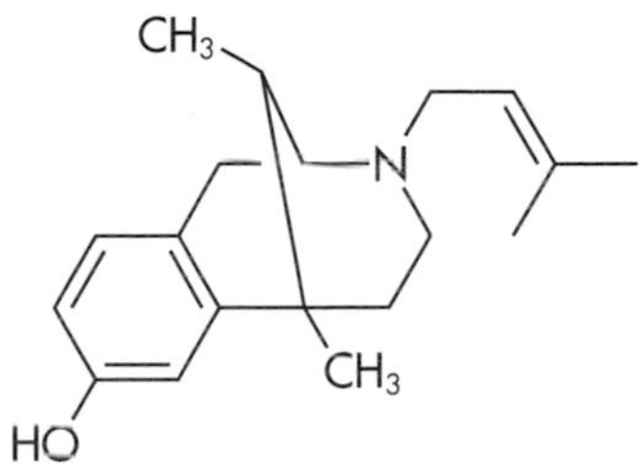

Pentazocine structure with CH₃, N, CH₃ and HO

	Pathway
Cocaine	Hydrolysis of methyl ester
	Hydrolysis of benzoate ester
	N-dealkylation
	Both hydrolysis and N-dealkylation

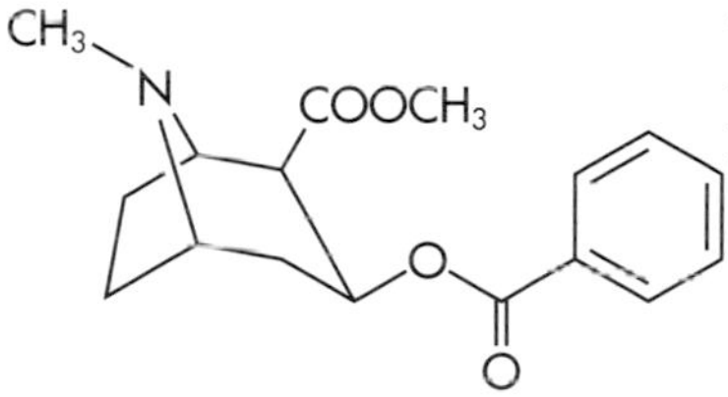

Cocaine structure with CH₃, N, COOCH₃

	Pathway
Phenmetrazine	Oxidation to lactam
	Aromatic hydroxylation
	N-oxidation
	Conjugation of phenolic products

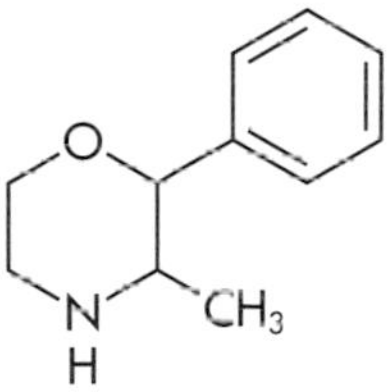

Phenmetrazine structure with O, N, H, CH₃

	Pathway
Ephedrine	N-dealkylation
	Oxidative deamination
	Oxidation of deaminated product to benzoic acid
	Reduction of deaminated product to 1,2-diol

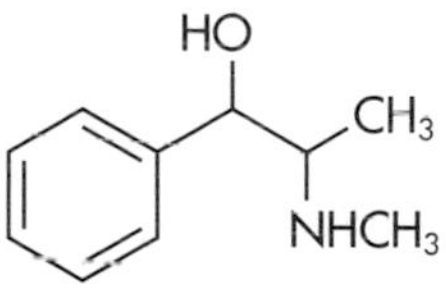

Ephedrine structure with HO, CH₃, NHCH₃

(continued)

Table 5.2 *Continued*

Drug	*Pathway*
Propranolol	Aromatic hydroxylation at C-4′
	N-dealkylation
	Oxidative deamination
	Oxidative of deaminated product to naphthoxylactic acid
	Conjugation with glucuronic acid
	O-dealkylation

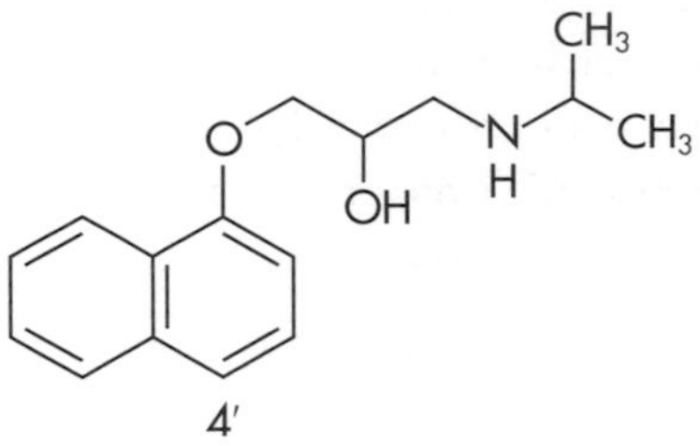

Indometacin	O-demethylation
	N-deacylation of p-chlorobenzoyl group
	Both O-dealkylation and N-deacylation
	Conjugation of phenolic products with glucuronic acid
	Other conjugation products

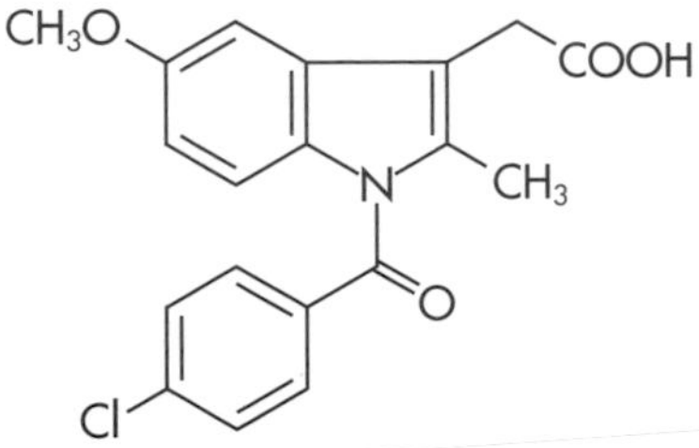

Diphenoxylate	Hydrolysis of ester to acid
	Hydroxylation of one aromatic ring attached to the N-alkyl side-chain

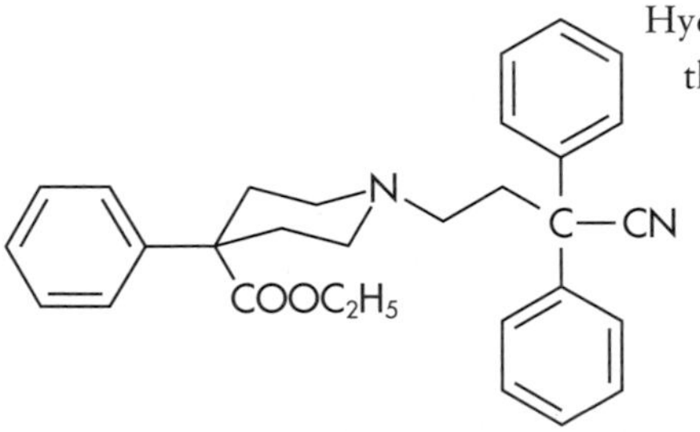

Diazepam	N-dealkylation at N^1
	Hydroxylation at carbon-3
	Conjugation of phenolic products with glucuronic acid
	Both N-dealkylation of N^1 and hydroxylation at carbon-3

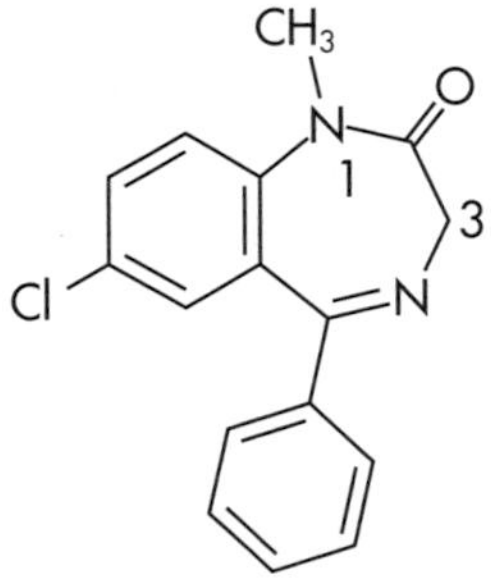

(*continued*)

Table 5.2 *Continued*

Drug	*Pathway*
Prostaglandins	Reduction of double bonds at carbons 5 and 6, and 13 and 14

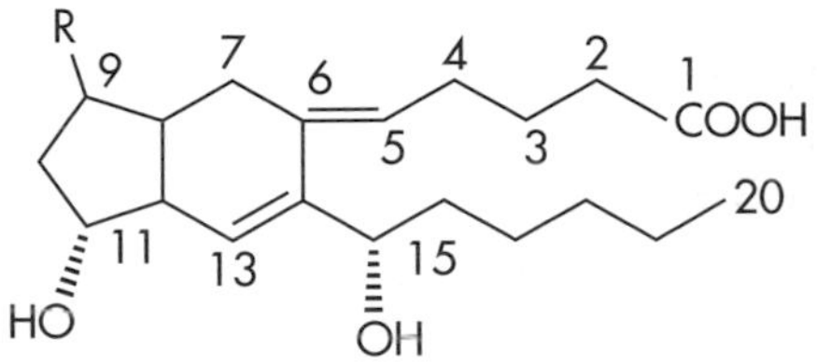

Oxidation of 15-hydroxyl to ketone
β-Oxidation of carbons 1, 2, 3 and 4
ω-Oxidation of carbon-20 to acid

Cyproheptadine

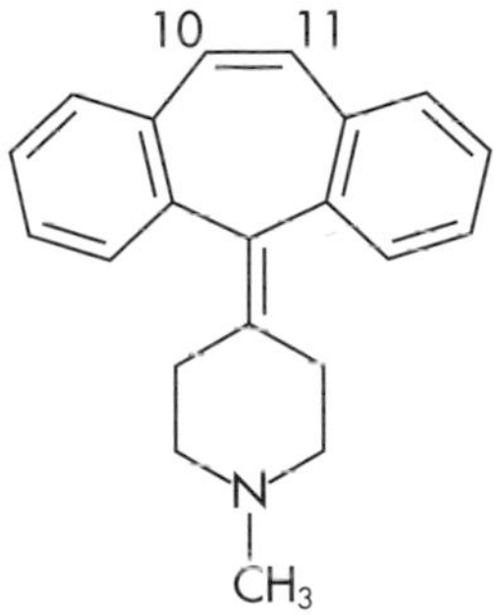

N-dealkylation
10,11-Epoxide formation
Both N-dealkylation and 10,11-epoxidation

Hydralazine

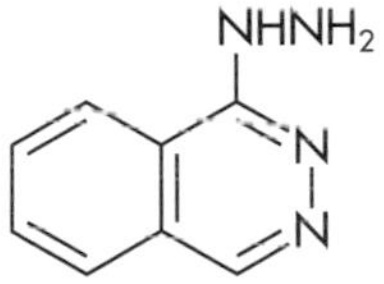

N-acetylation with cyclisation to a
   methyl-s-triazolophthalazine
N-formylation with cyclisation to an
   s-triazolophthalazine
Aromatic hydroxylation of benzene ring
Oxidative loss of hydrazinyl group to
   1-hydroxy
Hydroxylation of methyl of
   methyl-s-triazolophthalazine
Conjugation with glucuronic acid

Methadone

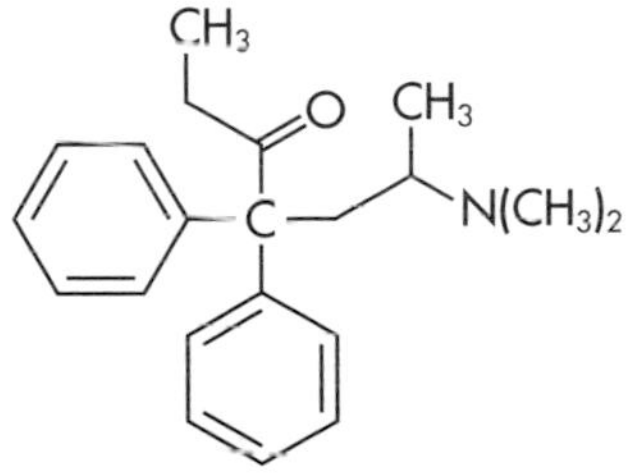

Reduction of ketone to hydroxyl
Aromatic hydroxylation of one aromatic ring
N-dealkylation of alcohol product
N-dealkylation with cyclisation to pyrrolidine

(continued)

Table 5.2 *Continued*

Drug	Pathway
Lidocaine (lignocaine)	*N*-dealkylation
	Oxidative cyclisation to a 4-imidazolidone
	N-oxidation of amide N
	Aromatic hydroxylation *ortho* to methyl
	Hydrolysis of amide

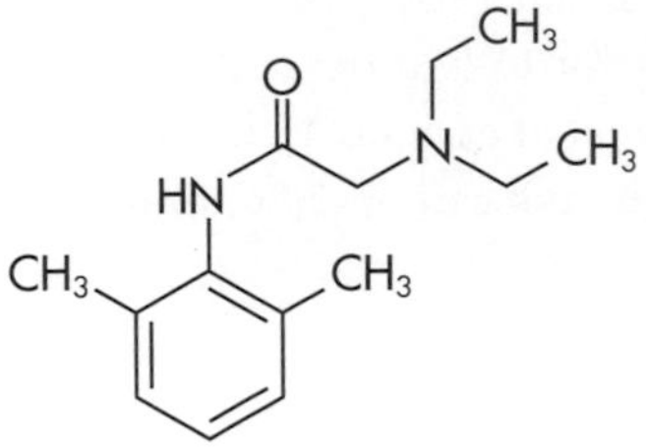

Drug	Pathway
Imipramine	*N*-dealkylation
	Hydroxylation at C-11
	Aromatic hydroxylation (C-2)
	N-oxidation
	Both *N*-dealkylation and hydroxylation

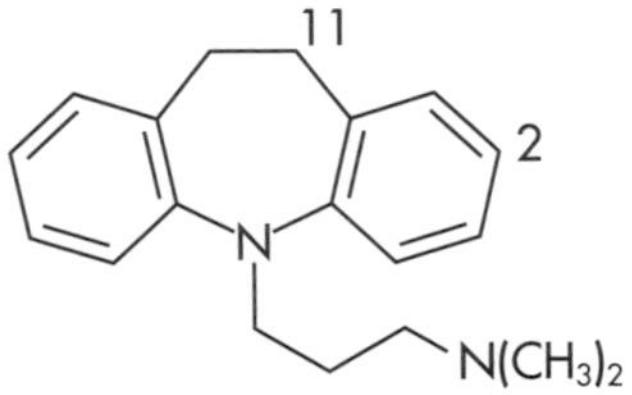

Drug	Pathway
Cimetidine	*S*-oxidation
	Hydroxylation of 5-methyl

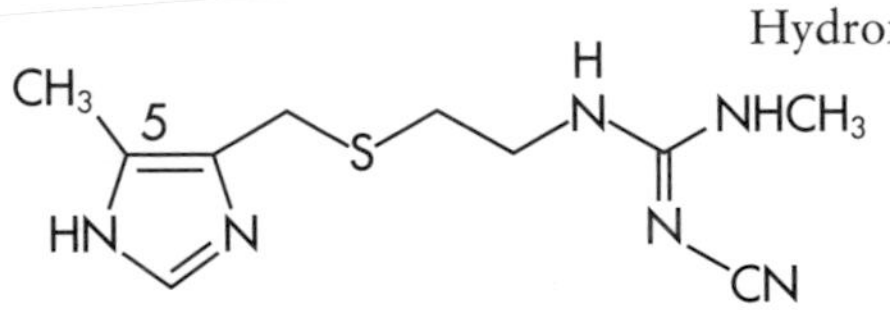

Drug	Pathway
Terfenadine	*N*-demethylation
	Methyl hydroxylation to CH_2OH
	CH_2OH oxidation to COOH

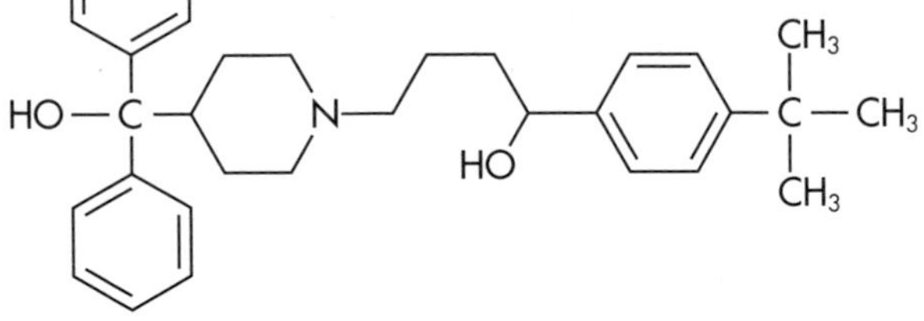

Drug	Pathway
Valproic Acid	CoA thioester
	Dehydrogenation to (*E*) 2-ene
	Dehydrogenation to (*E*) 2,4-diene
	Dehydrogenation to 4-ene
	3-Hydroxylation

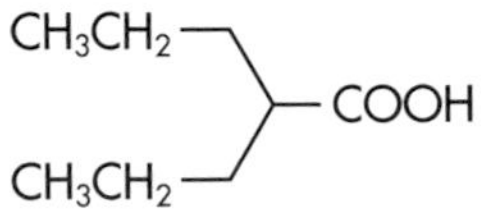

(*continued*)

Table 5.2   *Continued*

Drug	*Pathway*
Piroxicam	Pyridine 3'-hydroxylation
	Hydrolysis of amide
	Decarboxylation

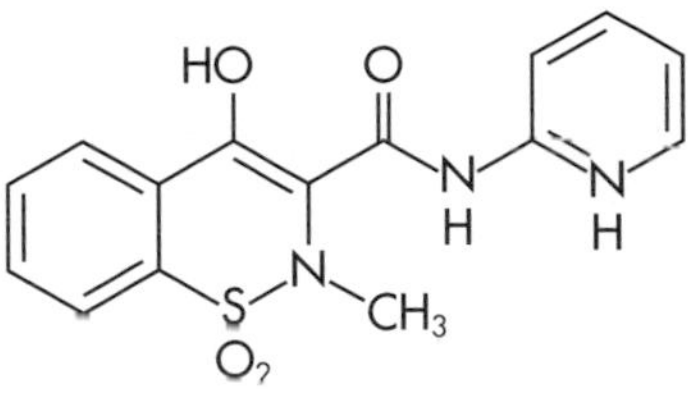

Caffeine	N^3-demethylation
	N^1-demethylation
	N^7-demethylation to theophylline
	C-8 oxidation to uric acids
	Imidazole ring opened

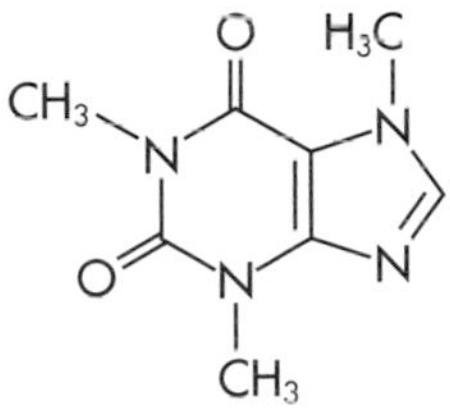

Theophylline	N^3-demethylation
	N^1-demethylation
	C-8 oxidation to uric acids
	1-methyl-xanthine to 1-methyl-uric acid with
	xanthine oxidase
	Imidazole ring opened

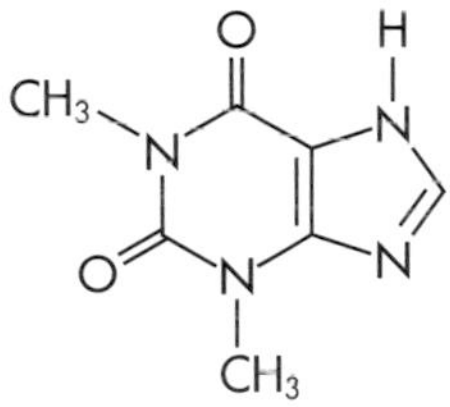

Nicotine	Pyrrolidine 5'-hydroxylation to cotinine
	Pyrrolidine N-oxidation (FMO)
	N-demethylation (nornicotine and norcotinine)
	Pyridine N-methylation
	3'-Hydroxylation of cotinine

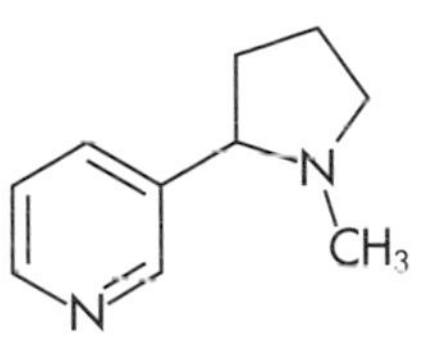

Ibuprofen	CoA thioester and epimerisation of (R)-(−) to
	(S)-(+)-enantiomer
	Methyl hydroxylation to CH_2OH
	CH_2OH to COOH
	Acylglucuronide

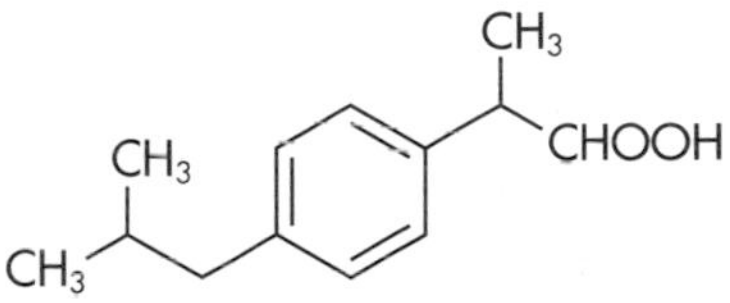

(*continued*)

Table 5.2 *Continued*

Drug	Pathway
Tamoxifen	N-demethylation
	4'-Hydroxylation
	N-Oxidation (FMO)
	4-O-sulfate
	4-O-glucuronide

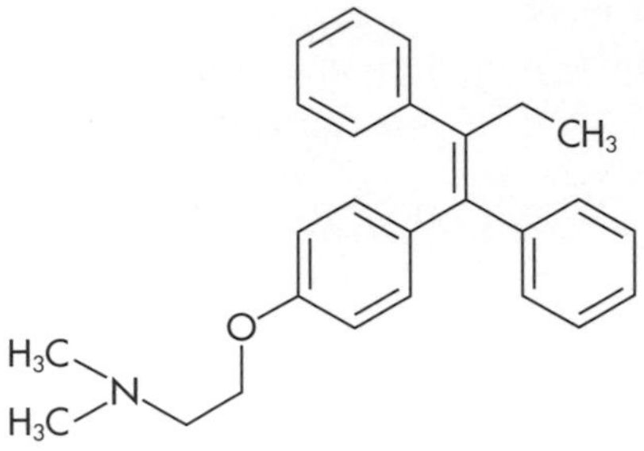

Lovastatin	6'-Hydroxylation
	3'-Side-chain hydroxylation
	3'-Hydroxylation
	β-Oxidation of lactone
	O-glucuronides

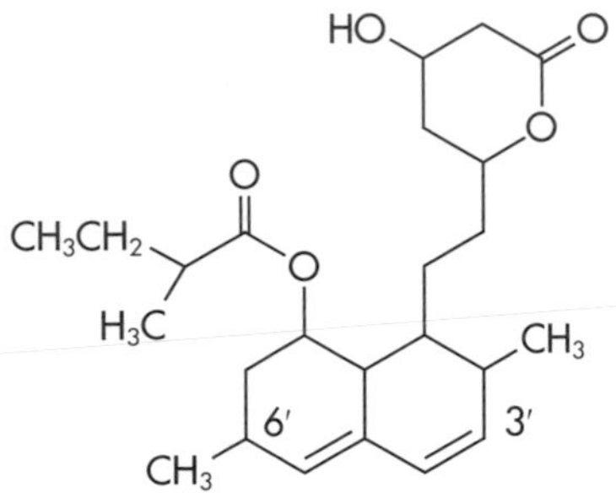

Ciprofloxacin	Piperazine 3'-hydroxylation
	N-sulfation

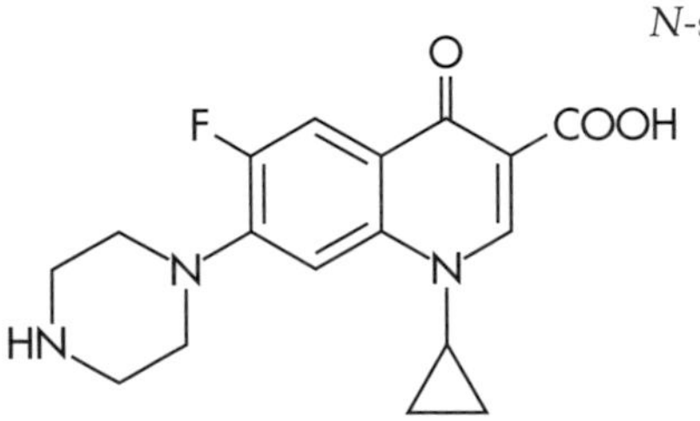

Labetalol	O-sulfate (major)
	O-glucuronide

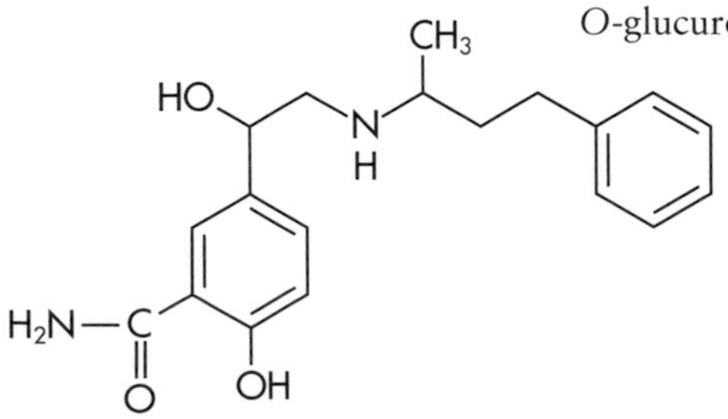

(*continued*)

Table 5.2   *Continued*

Drug	*Pathway*
Paracetamol	O-glucuronide
	O-sulfate
	Oxidation to N-acetyl-*p*-benzoquinoneimine
	Conjugation of N-acetyl-*p*-benzoquinoneimine
	with glutathione`

Tripelennamine	*p*-Hydroxylation
	Benzylic C-hydroxylation
	N-depyridinylation
	N-debenzylation

Felodipine	Aromatisation
	Ester hydrolysis
	Methyl hydroxylation

Tutorial example

 Explain why the insecticide malathion (Figure 5.9) is toxic to insects but relatively non-toxic to humans.

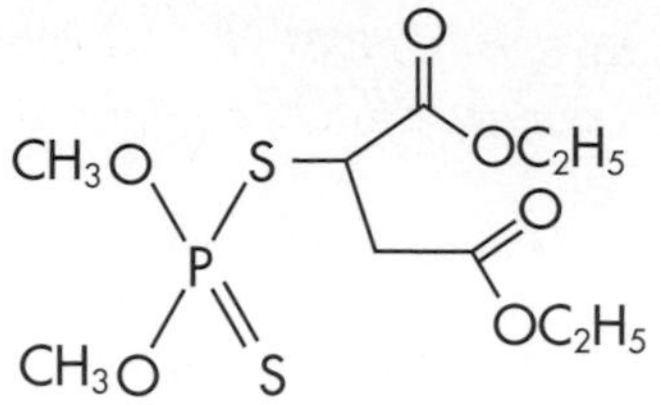

Figure 5.9 The structure of malathion.

 Malathion is an example of an organophosphorus insecticide, which works by inhibition of the enzyme acetylcholinesterase, responsible for the hydrolysis of the neurotransmitter acetylcholine. Inhibition of the enzyme allows the build-up of lethal concentrations of acetylcholine, convulsions and death. Malathion is a weak inhibitor of the enzyme and in humans is hydrolysed to the corresponding acid, which also has a low biological activity. In insects, malathion is oxidised to malaoxon which is 10 000 times more active than the parent

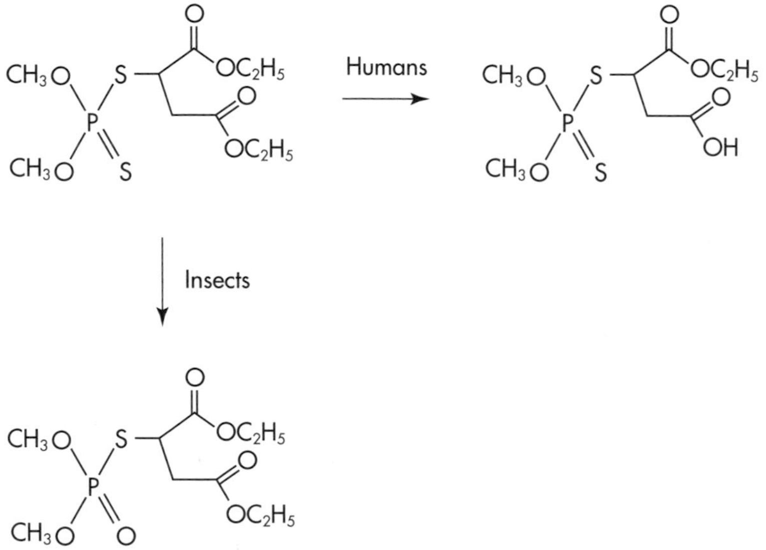

Humans

Insects

Figure 5.10 The metabolism of malathion.

compound. This results in an increase in levels of acetylcholine, which kills the insect (see Figure 5.10).

This example illustrates two important points. First, malathion is a selectively toxic compound in that it kills insects without harming humans. Second, different species may metabolise drugs in different ways and extreme care must be exercised when extrapolating results from one species to another, notably from animal toxicity data to humans.

Problems

Q5.1   The primary metabolic step involves a different mechanism for each of the drugs listed in Figure 5.11. Select the appropriate

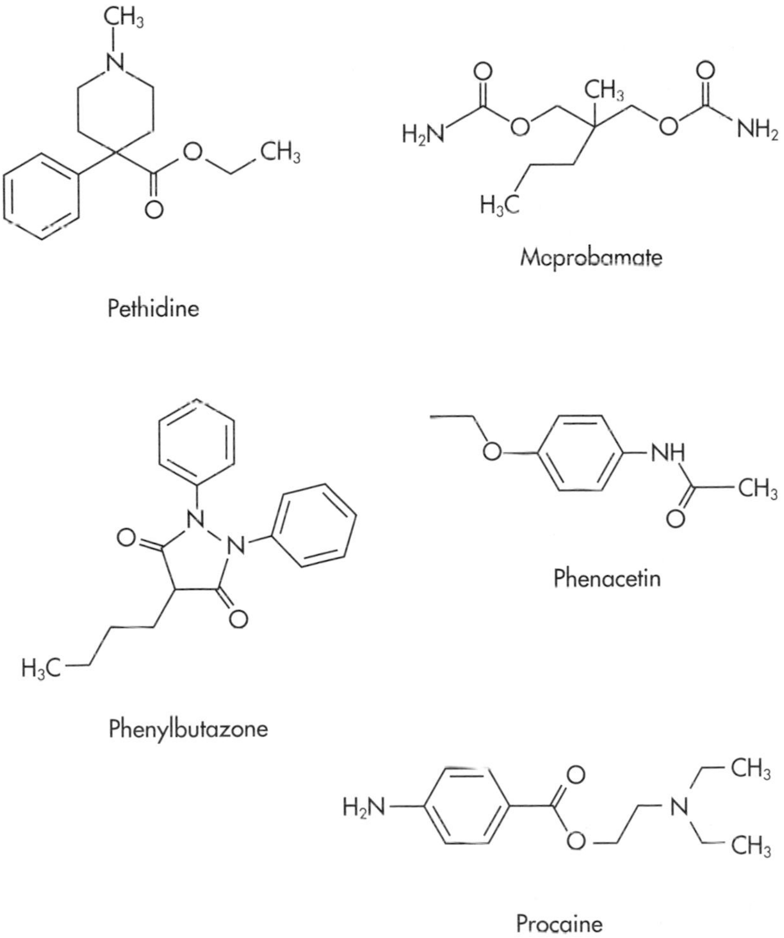

Pethidine

Meprobamate

Phenylbutazone

Phenacetin

Procaine

Figure 5.11   The structures of the drugs in Q5.1.

transformation for each drug from the following list: *aliphatic hydroxylation, oxidative N-dealkylation, hydrolysis, aromatic hydroxylation, oxidative O-dealkylation.* Draw the structure of the primary metabolite in each case.

Q5.2 Reactions that metabolically modify drugs and other xenobiotics are sometimes classified as Phase 1 and Phase 2 reactions. Explain the difference(s) between these two processes and give an example of each type of metabolism.

(Answers to problems may be found on pp. 221–222.)

6

Volumetric analysis of drugs

This chapter will deal with *volumetric analysis*, that is analysis carried out by the accurate measurement of volumes. To measure volumes accurately, use must be made of volumetric glassware. There are three pieces of volumetric glassware that are fundamental to successful volumetric analysis. These are the *volumetric flask*, the *pipette* and the *burette*, and each will be described below (see Figure 6.1). It should be stated, however, that no amount of reading about these pieces of apparatus (no matter how eloquently written!) is sufficient to educate a student. Analytical pharmaceutical chemistry is first and foremost a practical subject, and the laboratory is the best place to get to grips with the techniques required for consistent, reproducible analysis.

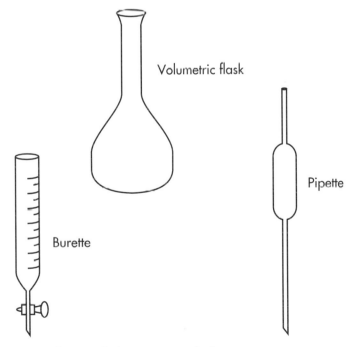

Figure 6.1 A volumetric flask, a pipette and a burette.

Volumetric flask

A volumetric flask is used to prepare accurate volumes of solution. These flasks are pear-shaped with long thin necks that allow the operator to dilute accurately to the mark with solvent. Volumetric flasks are available in all sizes from 1 mL up to 10 litres, but the most common sizes are 20, 50 and 100 mL. When selecting which size of flask to use, a compromise should be reached between the desire to use a small-volume flask and so save on expensive reagent, and the desire to use a large-volume flask to minimise dilution errors. The usual procedure is to pipette in a known volume of concentrated solution, add solvent until just short of the mark, shake or invert the flask to mix the contents and then make up to the mark, as accurately as possible, with a Pasteur pipette. Volumetric flasks should be used for all accurate dilutions. Use of measuring cylinders or (even worse) beakers to dilute solutions should be avoided.

Pipette

Pipettes are used to transfer accurate volumes of solution from a container (usually a beaker) to a reaction flask for dilution or assay, usually in conjunction with pipette fillers. They are not drinking straws and should never be placed in the mouth, or used to 'mouth pipette' solutions. This practice is both dangerous and unhygienic. There are two main types of pipettes.

Transfer (or delivery) pipettes

Pipettes of this type possess only one graduation mark and are used for delivery of that single volume of solution. Common sizes are 10, 20 and 50 mL. These pipettes are filled to a little above the mark by use of a pipette pump or a bulb. The pump is removed and the solution is allowed to run out until the mark is reached, the flow of solution being controlled all the way by use of the index finger over the end of the pipette. Most transfer pipettes are calibrated to allow a small volume of solution to remain in the tip of the pipette once it has been drained and no attempt should be made to 'blow' this drop out of the bottom of the pipette. Pipettes of this type are used in all analytical chemistry procedures.

Care must be taken when inserting the pipette into the pipette filler. If the pipette is held by the bulb and pushed into the filler, the shaft of the pipette can break and the operator can be injured. When inserting pipettes into pipette fillers, the pipette must always be held close to the end to prevent this all too common accident occurring.

Graduated pipettes

Graduated pipettes are calibrated to allow a single piece of glassware to deliver a range of volumes, common sizes are 1 mL and 10 mL. These pipettes are considerably less accurate than transfer pipettes, and there is no place for them in an analytical chemistry laboratory. If very small volumes need to be transferred, use should be made of accurate glass syringes (e.g. a 'Hamilton' syringe) or an automatic micropipette.

Burettes

Burettes are used to deliver variable volumes of reagent accurately. The most useful size is the 50 mL burette. These burettes are calibrated in units of 0.1 mL, but students should be encouraged to read to the nearest 0.05 mL. Once students have achieved some skill in titration techniques, they will be able to read the burette to the nearest 0.02 mL. This will involve splitting each 0.1 mL graduation into five – i.e. 0.02, 0.04, 0.06, 0.08 and 0.1 mL.

All of the volumetric glassware described above is designed for use at ambient room temperature and should never be used for hot liquids or placed in hot ovens and the like to dry.

Units of concentration

Before we consider topics such as the design of an assay, calculation of drug purity, and so on, it is useful to revise the units and terms chemists use for amount of substance and concentration. The fundamental unit of quantity or amount of substance used in chemistry is the *mole*. The mole is the amount of a substance (either elements or compounds) that contains the same number of atoms or molecules as there are in 12.0000 g of carbon-12. This number is known as the Avogadro number, or Avogadro's constant, and has the value 6.02×10^{23}. When this amount of substance is dissolved in solvent (usually water) and made up to 1 litre, a 1 molar (1 M) solution is produced. In a similar way, if one mole of substance were made up to 2 litres of solvent, a 0.5 M solution would result, and so on. The litre is not the SI unit of volume but, along with the millilitre (mL), is still used in the British Pharmacopoeia.

In pharmaceutical analysis laboratories, concentration is usually expressed as (for example) 1 M (1.026) or 0.5 M (0.998). The nominal concentration is given as molarity, while the number in brackets refers to the *factor* (f) of the solution. The factor of a volumetric solution tells you by how much the given solution differs from the nominal, or desired strength. The first solution, above, is slightly stronger than 1 M, since the factor is greater than 1.000. The second solution is slightly weaker than half molar, as the factor is less than 1.000. It follows that a solution with a factor of 1.000 is of precisely the stated molarity.

If the absolute molarity of the solution is required, it can easily be found by multiplying the factor and the nominal molarity. For instance, in the examples above, the first solution has an absolute molarity of 1 M × 1.026 = 1.026 M, which as predicted above is slightly stronger than 1 M. Similarly, the second solution has an absolute molarity of 0.499 M (i.e. 0.5 M × 0.998). It follows from this that the factor of a solution is simply the ratio

$$\frac{\text{Actual concentration}}{\text{Desired or nominal concentration}}$$

Factors are used in volumetric analysis because they simplify calculations (a laudable aim, in any subject). Consider the first solution above: the strength of the solution is 1 M (1.026). If 10 mL of this solution were removed, by pipette, transferred to a 100 mL volumetric flask, and made up to volume with water, the resulting solution would have a concentration of 0.1 M (1.026). The original solution has been diluted tenfold, but the factor of the new solution remains as 1.026. This illustrates an important principle, namely, that once a factor has been determined for a volumetric solution, subsequent dilution or reaction will not affect it (although see later for an exception to this).

Once the factor for a solution is known (i.e. once the solution has been *standardised*), multiplication of the experimentally determined volume by the factor will yield what the volume would have been if the solution had been precisely the nominal molarity (i.e. if the factor had been 1.000). In practice, very few volumetric solutions are factor 1.000, this is due, in the main, to the time that would be taken to weigh out a sample to four decimal places. Volumetric solutions are usually prepared by weighing out approximately the desired weight of sample, then standardising the resulting solution against a solution of known concentration.

All volumetric solutions used in pharmaceutical analysis are prepared from a *primary standard*. This is a compound that can be obtained in a very high level of purity (>99.9%). Examples of compounds used as primary standards include sodium carbonate (Na_2CO_3) and potassium hydrogen phthalate ($C_8H_5O_4K$). Compounds such as these can be weighed accurately, to four or even six decimal places, and made up to volume in a volumetric flask, to give a solution of known molarity. Solutions that are prepared by standardisation against a primary standard are referred to as secondary standards. A solution standardised against a secondary standard is termed a tertiary standard, and so on. This process cannot continue indefinitely, however, as errors creep in with every assay, and the results become less reliable the farther the solution gets from the initial primary standard.

Worked example

A primary standard solution of Na_2CO_3 was prepared and used to standardise a solution of H_2SO_4 of unknown concentration. 25.0 mL of 1 M ($f = 1.000$) Na_2CO_3 was added by pipette to a conical flask and 24.60 mL of H_2SO_4 was required for neutralisation. Calculate the factor of the H_2SO_4 solution.

From the reaction

$$Na_2CO_3 + H_2SO_4 \rightarrow Na_2SO_4 + CO_2 + H_2O$$

it can be seen that 1 mole of sodium carbonate reacts with 1 mole of sulfuric acid. Then

$$1 \text{ mole } Na_2CO_3 \equiv 1 \text{ mole } H_2SO_4$$

$$1000 \text{ mL } 1 \text{ M } Na_2CO_3 \equiv 1000 \text{ mL } 1 \text{ M } H_2SO_4$$

$$1 \text{ mL } 1 \text{ M } Na_2CO_3 \equiv 1 \text{ mL } 1 \text{ M } H_2SO_4$$

Since both solutions are 1 M, the concentrations effectively cancel out to leave the relationship

$$(\text{volume} \times \text{factor}) \text{ of } Na_2CO_3 = (\text{volume} \times \text{factor}) \text{ of } H_2SO_4$$

or, to put it another way,

$$(25 \text{ mL} \times f(Na_2CO_3)) \equiv (24.60 \text{ mL} \times f(H_2SO_4))$$

$$(25 \text{ mL} \times 1.000) \equiv (24.60 \text{ mL} \times f(H_2SO_4))$$

and $f(H_2SO_4)$ is given by $25 \times \dfrac{1.000}{24.6}$, so that

$$f(H_2SO_4) = 1.016$$

A moment's thought will confirm that the correct answer has been achieved. The only calculation error that could be made in this simple example is to get the factor upside-down (a so called 'inverted factor'). But, in the reaction, 25 mL of a $f = 1.000$ solution of Na_2CO_3 was neutralised by *less than* 25 mL of the acid. The acid must clearly be stronger than $f = 1.000$ if it required only 24.60 mL to neutralise the 25 mL of sodium carbonate. A check of this type should be carried out after every volumetric calculation. It is quick and easy to do and, to paraphrase the great Robert Burns, 'It wad frae monie a blunder free us, An' foolish notion.'

Concentration of active ingredients

Although, in chemistry, all concentrations are expressed in molarity, pharmacists and pharmaceutical analysts have to contend with the medical profession, which tends to prescribe drugs not in molarities but in units of mass per volume or weight per millilitre. The most common way to express the concentration of active drug in a medicine is in terms of mass or volume of active ingredient per 100 grams or millilitres of medicine. This can be expressed in four ways, of which the first is the most common.

- 'Percentage weight in volume' (% w/v) is the number of grams of drug in 100 mL of final product. This term is used for the concentrations of solutions, suspensions, etc. where the active ingredient is a solid; for example, 5% dextrose infusion is 5 g of dextrose in 100 mL of final solution.
- 'Percentage volume in volume' (% v/v) is the number of millilitres of drug in 100 mL of final product. This version is found in medicines where the active drug and the final product are both liquids. This terminology should be familiar to students since the strength of alcoholic drinks is usually expressed in this way. A single malt whisky is 40% by volume alcohol. This means that for every 100 mL of 'Glen Whatever' you drink you consume 40 mL of ethanol. Most beers are approximately 5% by volume alcohol. Thus, for every 100 mL of beer consumed, the drinker has taken in 5 mL of ethanol. (A pint is approximately 568 mL.)
- 'Percentage weight in weight' (% w/w) is the number of grams of drug in 100 g of final product. This term is encountered most often in solid dosage preparations such as powders, and semi-solid preparations such as creams and ointments, e.g. 1% salicylic acid ointment.
- 'Percentage volume in weight' (% v/w) is the number of millilitres of drug in 100 g of final product. This usage is quite rare and is only encountered in ointments and creams where the active ingredient is a liquid, e.g. 1% glycerol ointment.

Design of an assay

Before a substance is analysed, or assayed, the experiment must be designed and planned. Initially, students will be told what to do in the analysis laboratory, but they must quickly begin to plan assays and experiments for themselves. The procedures to be followed when designing an assay are outlined below.

1. Identify functional groups on the molecule that can react rapidly and quantitatively (i.e. the reaction should proceed almost 100% to the products; to put it another way, the chosen reaction should have a high equilibrium constant, K).

2. Work out the stoichiometric ratio, i.e. the number of moles of each compound reacting.

3. Convert the number of moles of sample to a weight, and the number of moles of titrant to a volume.

4. Calculate the weight of sample that will react with 1 mL of the titrant. This figure is called the *equivalent relationship* or sometimes *the equivalent* and is the most important part of the calculation.

5. Carry out the assay, at least in duplicate. If agreement is not achieved with two results, the assay should be repeated until concordant results are obtained.

6. Calculate the weight of active drug in the sample, and express the answer as percentage weight in weight (% w/w) of sample weighed. This answer represents the percentage purity of the drug and should be compared to the *British Pharmacopoeia* (BP) limits to see whether the sample complies with the requirements of the BP. The *British Pharmacopoeia* lays down purity criteria and limits within which a sample must lie to be of BP quality. Both determinations must fall within the BP limits to be acceptable. If one result falls within the BP limits and the duplicate result does not, then the sample does not comply with the BP limits, and should not be used.

In addition to the limits of purity, the British Pharmacopoeia contains a wealth of information about the substance in question. The *British Pharmacopoeia* is a legally enforceable document produced every four or five years by the Pharmacopoeia Commission and lists the criteria for the purity of drugs and medicines used in the UK and Commonwealth. Each substance in the *British Pharmacopoeia* is given a specific *monograph*, which lists the chemical structure of the compound (if known), the definition and statement of BP limits (quoted to one decimal place), a description of its characteristics (colour, solubility, etc.), some tests for identification of a sample of the material and limit tests for impurities (usually a colour test that compares the levels of an impurity with the maximum permitted limit allowed by the BP for that impurity). Limit tests are often used when the BP assay is not *stability indicating*, i.e. does not differentiate between the drug and its major decomposition product. The monograph ends with the official BP assay for determination of purity. Formulated medicines may have, in addition to a specific monograph, a *general monograph*, which applies to that class of medicine. For example Aspirin Tablets BP will have to comply with all of the monograph for Aspirin BP as well as the general monograph for *tablets*. Similarly, Chloramphenicol Eye Drops BP must comply with the general monograph on *eye drops* for sterility, etc. in addition to the requirements for the purity of chloramphenicol.

To illustrate these points, we can consider the assay of citric acid. Citric acid is a natural product found in citrus fruits (lemons, oranges, limes, etc.) and is used in pharmaceutical formulations as a buffer and a preservative. Its structure is shown in Figure 6.2.

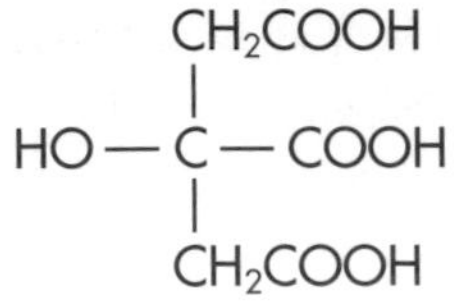

$$
\begin{array}{c}
CH_2COOH \\
|\\
HO-C-COOH \\
|\\
CH_2COOH
\end{array}
$$

Figure 6.2   The structure of citric acid.

Examination of the structure of citric acid reveals three carboxylic acid groups; these should react quantitatively with a strong alkali, such as sodium hydroxide. So the reaction equation is

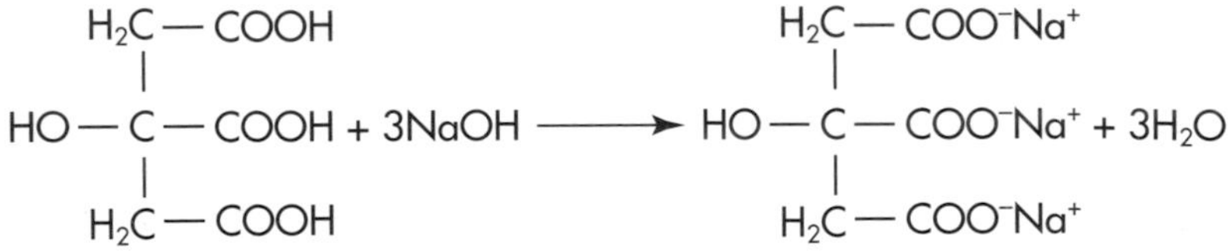

$$
\begin{array}{c}
H_2C-COOH \\
|\\
HO-C-COOH + 3NaOH \\
|\\
H_2C-COOH
\end{array}
\longrightarrow
\begin{array}{c}
H_2C-COO^-Na^+ \\
|\\
HO-C-COO^-Na^+ + 3H_2O \\
|\\
H_2C-COO^-Na^+
\end{array}
$$

Therefore,

1 mole citric acid $\equiv$ 3 moles NaOH

and

192.1 g citric acid $\equiv$ 3 litres 1 M NaOH

or

192.1 g citric acid $\equiv$ 3000 mL 1 M NaOH

Therefore,

(192.1/3000) g citric acid $\equiv$ 1 mL 1 M NaOH

or

0.06403 g citric acid $\equiv$ 1 mL 1 M NaOH

The equation in bold type is the equivalent relationship and tells us that for every 1 mL of titrant added, we can expect to react slightly more than 64 mg of citric acid. Note also that the equivalent is derived for a precisely 1 M solution, i.e. $f = 1.000$.

This reaction was carried out using phenolphthalein as an indicator and the following data were obtained.

Weight of citric acid = 1.5268 g

Volume of 1 M NaOH ($f = 0.998$) required 23.95 mL

The volume of titrant used in the assay must now be modified to give what the volume would have been if a factor 1.000 solution had been used. This is achieved by multiplying the experimental volume by the factor, so that

23.95 ml of titrant ($f = 0.998$)

$\equiv (23.95 \times 0.998)$ ml 1 NaOH ($f = 1.000$)

Since, from the equivalent,

1 mL 1 M NaOH ($f = 1.000$) $\equiv 0.06403$ g citric acid

then the weight of citric acid in the sample is given by

$(23.95 \times 0.998 \times 0.06403)$ g

However, 1.5268 g was weighed, so the content of citric acid is given by

$$\frac{23.95 \times 0.998 \times 0.06403}{1.5268} = 1.0024$$

This figure is usually expressed as a percentage, to give the percentage purity of citric acid as 100.2% w/w.

A duplicate determination is now carried out and the answer compared to 100.2% w/w. Agreement is usually considered to be not more than 0.5% error between duplicates. Once duplicate determinations have been carried out, and agreement is obtained, the answers may be averaged and the *British Pharmacopoeia* consulted to see whether the sample complies. Not every sample assayed will comply; there may be impurities present if, for example, the sample was old or had been adulterated. However, an analyst who has obtained duplicate results, in good agreement, should be confident to state that the sample does not comply with the BP limits.

Practical points

Weighing by difference

In all accurate pharmaceutical analyses, samples are weighed by difference, that is the weight of sample added to the flask is determined by subtraction of consecutive weighings of the sample container. The procedure adopted is as follows.

1. Twice the desired amount of sample is weighed roughly on a top pan balance (i.e. if a procedure requires a sample weight of 1.5 g, then for duplicate determinations 2 × 1.5 g = 3.0 g will be required).

2. The sample container and contents are weighed accurately on an analytical balance, to four, or sometimes six, decimal places.

3. Some of the sample is transferred to the reaction flask and the sample container is re-weighed. Care should be taken not to touch the sample with the fingers, a spatula, or anything else for that matter. The difference in weight between steps 2 and 3 represents the weight of sample transferred.

4. This process is repeated until the desired weight has been transferred. If more than the desired weight of sample is transferred, the sample should be discarded and the whole procedure begun again. *On no account should excess sample be returned to the original container.* The *British Pharmacopoeia* allows discretion of ±10% on the stated sample weights.

Approximate titre calculation

The end point of a titration should not come as a surprise to the analyst. Before a single drop of titrant has been added, an estimate of the end-point volume should be carried out. For a simple forward titration, like the citric acid example above, the approximate titre is given by

$$\frac{\text{Sample weight}}{\text{Equivalent weight}} = x \text{ mL}$$

This calculation makes two assumptions, neither of which is actually valid, namely that the factor of the titrant to be used in the assay is 1.000, and that the sample is 100% pure. Neither of these assumptions will be true, but the factor will be close to 1.000 and the purity will, usually, be close to 100%, so the estimate is worth doing. The approximate titre calculation is also the first sign the analyst has that things are going wrong in the assay. If the approximate titre is estimated as (say) 18 mL, alarm bells should begin to ring if no end point has been reached after approximately 20 mL. The stated sample weights in the BP are usually chosen to give titres between 20 and 25 mL. This is because analysts are, by nature, lazy and do not want to have to refill a 50 mL burette during a titration!

Use of molarities in calculation

Students often prefer to perform simple calculations, like the direct titration of citric acid, using absolute molarities of titrant instead of deriving the equivalent and making use of factors. This view is shared by some colleagues (particularly those from a pure chemistry background).

The procedure adopted is to convert the volume of titrant required to a number of moles and, from the balanced chemical equation, relate this to the number of moles of reactant used in the assay. This number

Indicator	pH 1	2	3	4	5	6	7	8	9	10	11	12	13
Cresol Red	Red	Orange			Yellow				Pink	Red			
Metacresol Purple	Red	Orange			Yellow				Grey	Violet			
Tropaeolin OO	Red	Orange	Yellow										
Thymol Blue	Red	Orange				Yellow			Grey	Violet-blue			
Metanil Yellow	Red	Orange	Yellow										
Naphthol Yellow	Colourless	Pale Yellow	Yellow										
Bromophenol Blue		Yellow	Grey	Blue-violet									
Methyl Orange		Red	Orange	Yellow									
Methyl Orange-Xylene Cyanol FF		Violet	Grey	Green									
Dimethyl Yellow		Red	Orange	Yellow									
Congo Red		Blue	Violet	Red									
Bromocresol Green		Yellow	Green	Blue									
Methyl Red			Red	Orange	Yellow								
Litmus			Red	Violet	Blue								
Bromocresol Purple			Yellow	Grey	Blue-violet								
Bromothymol Blue			Yellow	Green	Blue								
Neutral Red				Red	Orange-red	Orange							
Phenol Red				Yellow	Pink	Red							
1- Naphtholphthalein				Pale red	Green	Blue							
Phenolphthalein					Colourless	Pink	Red						
Thymolphthalein					Colourless	Pale blue	Blue						
Alizarin Yellow GG					Colourless	Pale yellow	Yellow						
Tropaeolin O							Yellow	Yellow-orange	Orange				
Titan yellow							Yellow	Orange	Red				

Figure 6.3 A table of the pH ranges of indicators.

is then converted into a weight and the purity is obtained by dividing this calculated weight by the mass of sample weighed out. Sources of error can be introduced in each conversion from volume to moles and back to weight, although, for simple examples such as the one above it does not really matter which method of calculation is employed as long as the correct answer for the purity of citric acid is obtained. However, for more complicated calculations, involving the use of back and blank titrations, this author believes that factors and equivalents simplify volumetric analysis and they will be used for that reason (rather than any reason of dogma) in the remainder of this book.

Choice of indicators

The end point of the titration is detected by the use of a suitable indicator. These indicators are themselves weak acids or bases whose colour in solution depends on their degree of ionisation. In practice, the end-point pH is estimated (see Chapter 1, p. 20), and an indicator that changes colour at this pH chosen. For convenience, a table of common indicators and their pH ranges is shown in Figure 6.3.

Back and blank titrations

In the example above, a reaction was chosen that was quick to carry out and was quantitative, i.e. it went to completion. In many pharmaceutical analyses this is not the case and a *back titration* has to be carried out. Back titrations are often combined with *blank titrations*, particularly if there is some loss of reagent during the assay (e.g. as a result of splashing or vigorous boiling) or the concentration of a volumetric reagent changes during the assay.

A back titration involves addition of a known excess of reagent to the sample (this drives the reaction to completion) and titration of the unreacted excess of reagent with a suitable titrant. The volume that reacted with the sample is determined by simple subtraction. For example, if 50.0 mL of reagent were added to the sample and the back titre was 30.0 mL then, clearly, 20.0 mL of reagent has reacted with the sample.

In a blank titration, the assay is carried out, then repeated without any sample being present. This appears, at first sight, to be a perfect waste of time, but determinations of this type allow the analyst to measure any changes that occur to the reagent during the course of the assay. If the procedure involves heating and subsequent cooling of the sample (e.g. to allow the sample to dissolve), some of the volumetric reagent may be lost either by evaporation or mechanically due to splashing or bubbling. The blank determination must be identical to the test determination in every way except, of course, that there is no sample in the blank. This means that heating times, dilutions, etc. must all be duplicated exactly.

The best way to illustrate the procedures adopted for back and blank titrations is to consider an example, the determination of chalk, or calcium carbonate, $CaCO_3$. Chalk is used as an antacid and indigestion remedy, particularly in children, and is official in the *British Pharmacopoeia* as the powder and the mixture (Paediatric Chalk BP).

The official assay is by the addition of a known excess of hydrochloric acid and back titration of the unreacted excess with sodium hydroxide. A blank determination is carried out since the sample is heated and cooled. The calculation will be carried out initially as a back titration without a blank and then compared with the answer obtained when the blank is taken into account. The calculation should be studied closely as there are subtle differences between the back and blank calculations.

The chemical reactions taking place are as follows.

$$CaCO_3 + 2HCl \text{ (in excess)} \rightarrow CaCl_2 + CO_2 + H_2O$$

Then

$$2 \text{ HCl (unreacted excess)} + 2NaOH \rightarrow 2NaCl + 2H_2O$$

The relative molecular mass of chalk is 100.1, so that

$$1 \text{ mole } CaCO_3 \equiv 2 \text{ moles HCl} \equiv 2 \text{ moles NaOH}$$

Therefore,

$$100.1 \text{ g } CaCO_3 \equiv 2000 \text{ mL 1 M HCl}$$
$$\equiv 2000 \text{ mL 1 M NaOH}$$

and

$$0.05005 \text{ g } CaCO_3 \equiv 1 \text{ mL 1 M HCl}$$
$$\equiv 1 \text{ mL 1 M NaOH}$$

In the experiment, approximately 1.5 g of sample was weighed and added to 100 mL of water in a conical flask and 50.0 mL of 1 M hydrochloric acid was added by pipette. The mixture was boiled gently for 2 minutes and cooled and the unreacted HCl was titrated with 1 M NaOH using methyl orange as indicator. The entire procedure was repeated omitting the sample and the % w/w $CaCO_3$ in the sample was determined.

Results

>   Weight of chalk = 1.5961 g
>
>   Volume of 1 M ($f = 0.996$) HCl = 50.00 mL
>
>   Volume of 1 M ($f = 1.012$) NaOH = 18.50 mL

Since neither volumetric solution is factor 1.000, the experimental volumes must be modified by the factor to obtain the factor 1.000 volumes.

>   Volume of HCl available = (50.0×0.996)
>
>   Volume of NaOH in excess = (18.50×1.012)

Therefore, the volume reacting with chalk is given by

> $(50.0 \times 0.996) - (18.50 \times 1.012) = 31.08$ mL

From the equivalent,

>   1 mL 1 M HCl or NaOH $\equiv$ 0.05005 g $CaCO_3$

Therefore,

>   31.08 ml 1 M solution $\equiv (31.08 \times 0.05005)$ g $CaCO_3$ = 1.5554 g $CaCO_3$

However, 1.5931 g of sample was weighed. Therefore, the percentage of calcium carbonate is

$$\frac{1.5554}{1.5931} \times 100 = 97.6\% \text{ w/w}$$

Using these same data, the calculation can be repeated, but this time taking account of the blank determination. If an assay requires a blank, then the concentration of the reagent (hydrochloric acid in this case) must change in the course of the assay; therefore, the volume and factor of the hydrochloric acid will not appear anywhere in the calculation.

>   Volume of 1 M NaOH ($f = 1.012$) in blank titration $\approx$ 49.65 mL

In this case, the volume of 1 M NaOH reacting with chalk is given by

>   (Volume of blank titration – volume of back titration) × factor of NaOH

The NaOH factor is used because both of these volumes are NaOH volumes. That is,

> $(49.65 - 18.5) \times 1.012$ mL 1 M NaOH

Since from the equivalent

$$1 \text{ mL } 1 \text{ M NaOH} \equiv 0.05005 \text{ g CaCO}_3$$

then the weight of calcium carbonate in the sample is

$$(49.65 - 18.50) \times 1.012 \times 0.05005 \text{ g} = 1.5778 \text{ g CaCO}_3$$

However, 1.5931 g of chalk was weighed, so the percentage purity of calcium carbonate is

$$\frac{1.5778}{1.5931} \times 100 - 99.0\% \text{ w/w}$$

The calculation involving the blank should be more accurate than the back titration on its own since the NaOH has, in effect, been standardised during the course of the assay.

These two procedures should be studied closely since there is a subtle difference in calculation. In the back titration, the volume of acid was multiplied by the factor of the acid, and the volume of base was multiplied by the factor of the base. In the blank titration, neither the volume nor the factor of the reagent added in excess is required and the volume of titrant equivalent to the chalk is given by the expression (blank volume – test volume) × factor of titrant.

Assay of unit-dose medicines

Unit-dose medicines are preparations that contain doses designed to be taken separately. Examples of this type of preparation include tablets, capsules, suppositories or pessaries. To determine the purity of unit-dose medicines, the calculations outlined above need to be modified, in order to determine how much drug is present in each individual dosage form. The purity of the bulk powder sample is not so important. The drug content is expressed as a percentage of how much drug should be present and is called the *percentage of the stated amount*. The *British Pharmacopoeia* uses this calculation to express the purity of all unit-dose medicines.

An example of this type of calculation is the assay of Lithium Carbonate Tablets BP. Lithium carbonate is used as an antidepressant in 250 mg and 400 mg strengths. The BP assay is to weigh and powder 20 tablets. Add a quantity of the powder containing 1 g of lithium carbonate to 100 mL of water; add 50 mL of 1 M hydrochloric acid and boil for 1 minute to remove carbon dioxide. Cool and titrate the excess acid with 1 M sodium hydroxide solution using methyl orange as indicator.

The assay is then repeated omitting the sample.
The reactions taking place are as follows.

$$Li_2CO_3 + 2HCl \rightarrow 2LiCl + H_2O + CO_2$$
$$2HCl + 2NaOH \rightarrow 2NaCl + 2H_2O$$

Therefore, since the relative molecular mass of Li_2CO_3 is 73.9,

$$73.9 \text{ g } Li_2CO_3 \equiv 2000 \text{ mL 1 M NaOH}$$
$$0.03695 \text{ g } Li_2CO_3 \equiv 1 \text{ mL 1 M NaOH}$$

The assay was carried out and the following results were obtained.

Weight of 20 tablets = 3.7279 g

Weight of powder for assay = 0.4707 g

Volume of 1 M NaOH (f = 1.006) added (blank) = 48.75 mL

Volume of 1 M NaOH (f = 1.006) added (test) = 21.35 mL

The weight of 20 tablets is 3.7279 g; therefore, the average weight of one tablet is 3.7279/20 = 0.1864 g.
The weight of lithium carbonate in the sample is

$$(48.75 - 21.35) \times 1.006 \times 0.03695 \text{ g } Li_2CO_3$$
$$= 1.0185 \text{ g } Li_2CO_3$$

The number of tablets assayed is given by

$$\frac{\text{Sample weight}}{\text{Average weight of one tablet}}$$
$$= \frac{0.4707}{0.1864}$$
$$= 2.53 \text{ tablets}$$

Therefore, 1.0185 g lithium carbonate was found in 2.53 tablets, so the weight of lithium carbonate in one tablet is 1.0185/2.53 = 0.4034 g.
The stated content of lithium carbonate is 400 mg per tablet, so the percentage stated amount is given by (0.4034/0.4) × 100 = 100.8%.

Non-aqueous titrations

Non-aqueous titrations are titrations carried out in the absence of water. They are particularly useful for the assay of drugs that are very weakly acidic or basic, so weak in fact that they will not ionise in aqueous conditions. Water, being an amphoteric compound, acts to suppress the ionisation of very weak acids and bases. All the apparatus and glassware for a non-aqueous titration must be scrupulously dry, as even a drop of water will ruin the whole assay. All glassware should be rinsed with distilled water, rinsed again with a volatile solvent such as acetone, then dried thoroughly in an oven or hot air dryer. It is also a good idea to remove all wash bottles from the laboratory. There is no sadder sight than to watch a student conscientiously carry out a non-aqueous titration and then spoil all the hard work by thoughtlessly adding water from a wash bottle.

Non-aqueous titrations are widely used in Volume 1 of the *British Pharmacopoeia* for the assay of drug substances. A large number of drugs are either weakly acidic (such as barbiturates, phenytoin or sulfonamides), or weak bases (antihistamines, local anaesthetics, morphine, etc.). The weak acids are usually titrated with tetrabutylammonium hydroxide ($N(Bu^n)_4OH$) or potassium methoxide (CH_3OK) in dimethylformamide (DMF) as solvent. Weak bases are dissolved in glacial acetic acid and titrated with perchloric acid ($HClO_4$). When a strong acid, such as perchloric acid, is dissolved in a weaker acid, such as acetic acid, the acetic acid is forced to act as a base and accept a proton from the perchloric acid. This generates an *onium* ion, which functions, in the absence of water, as a super-strong acid, and it is this species that reacts with the basic drug.

The reactions occurring are as follows.

$$HClO_4 + CH_3COOH \rightarrow CH_3COOH_2^+ + ClO_4^-$$
$$CH_3COOH_2^+ + base \rightarrow CH_3COOH + base\ H^+$$

Overall, the reaction is

$$HClO_4 + base \rightarrow base\ H^+ + ClO_4^-$$

That is, the perchloric acid acts as a monoprotic acid and 1 mole of perchloric acid is equivalent to 1 mole of basic drug. The derivation of the equivalent and the calculations required are the same as for their aqueous counterparts.

REDOX titrations

REDOX titrations are titrations that involve the processes of *oxidation* and *reduction*. These two processes always occur together and are of huge importance in chemistry. Everything from simple ionic reactions to the generation of energy within human mitochondria depends on these two processes.

- Oxidation is defined as the loss of hydrogen, or the gain of oxygen, or the *loss of electrons*.

- Reduction is defined as the gain of hydrogen, or the loss of oxygen, or the *gain of electrons*.

In a REDOX titration, the equation for the reaction is balanced not by counting the moles of atoms reacting but rather by counting the moles of electrons transferred in the process. This can be illustrated by considering the standardisation of the common reagent potassium permanganate solution with the primary standard, oxalic acid. This natural compound can be obtained in high purity and is well-known in pharmacognosy as the toxic constituent of rhubarb leaves.

The reactions occurring are as follows.

$$MnO_4^- + 8H^+ + 5e^- \rightarrow Mn^{2+} + 4H_2O$$
$$(COOH)_2 \rightarrow 2CO_2 + 2H^+ + 2e^-$$

If the equation is balanced in terms of electrons:

$$2MnO_4^- (10e^-) \equiv 5(COOH)_2 (10e^-)$$
$$2000 \text{ mL 1 M } MnO_4^- \equiv 5 \times 126.1 \text{ g oxalic acid}$$
$$1 \text{ mL } 0.02 \text{ M } MnO_4^- \equiv 0.006305 \text{ g oxalic acid}$$

Other REDOX reagents include iodine (I_2), either by itself in a forward titration or in a back titration with sodium thiosulfate ($Na_2S_2O_3$), and complex salts of the metal cerium (such as ammonium cerium sulfate, $Ce(SO_4)_2 \cdot 2(NH_4)_2SO_4 \cdot 2H_2O$). Salts of this type are complex by name as well as by formula, but in reality behave as

$$Ce^{4+} + e^- \rightarrow Ce^{3+}$$

in solution. In the case of cerium, only one electron is transferred, and calculation of the equivalent relationship is very straightforward.

A good example of a back titration involving iodine and thiosulfate is the assay of resorcinol in Resorcinol Solution BP. Resorcinol is an antiseptic that was widely used in the past, although less so now. The assay of resorcinol involves a quantitative electrophilic aromatic substitution reaction using bromine as the reagent, as shown in Figure 6.4.

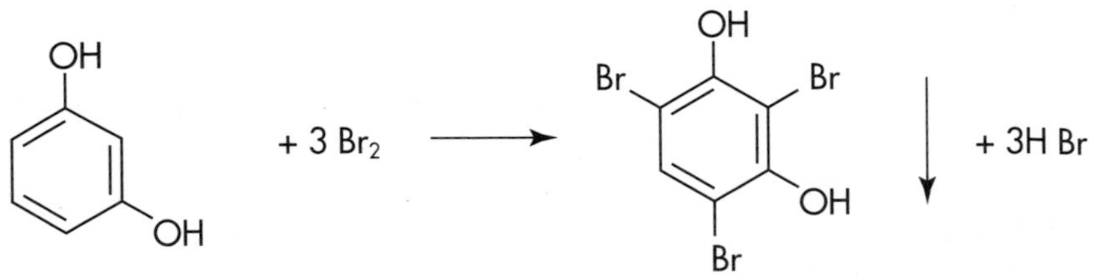

Figure 6.4   The reaction of resorcinol with bromine.

Bromine is a vapour at room temperature and pressure and so cannot be measured accurately by pipette. It is also an extremely corrosive compound, irritant to eyes, lungs and mucous membranes. To overcome these difficulties, the bromine required for reaction with the resorcinol is generated *in situ* by reaction of potassium bromate and potassium bromide in the presence of strong mineral acid.

$$KBrO_3^- + 5KBr + 6HCl \rightarrow 3Br_2 + 3H_2O + 6KCl$$

To ensure that the bromination reaction proceeds quantitatively to the right-hand side, an excess of bromine is generated and the volume of bromine that does not react with resorcinol is determined by back titration. Bromine cannot be titrated easily, so the excess bromine is determined by addition of an excess of potassium iodide and titration of the liberated iodine with sodium thiosulfate.

$$Br_2 + 2KI \rightarrow I_2 + 2KBr$$

$$I_2 + 2Na_2S_2O_3 \rightarrow 2NaI + S_4O_6$$

This assay is great fun to do because the whole titration is carried out using a special type of conical flask called an *iodine flask*. This type of flask has a glass well around the stopper into which the titrant is added. The stopper is then gently rotated (but not removed!) to allow titrant to enter. The iodine flask is used for two reasons:

- To prevent the escape of volatile bromine reagent
- To allow the contents to be shaken vigorously as the end point is approached

Some analysts choose to add a non-polar solvent such as chloroform to the reaction. The chloroform acts as a solvent for the iodine (which is not very soluble in water) and, by concentrating the colour in a small volume, increases the sensitivity of the assay. Often, a small amount of starch indicator is added (to the well of the flask) as the end point is approached. Starch forms a blue-black complex with iodine and the end point of the titration is reached when the blue colour in the chloroform has disappeared.

The calculation of the content of resorcinol in the solution is identical to the back titration method explained above for lithium carbonate. Consequently, the volume of added bromate is modified by the bromate factor and the thiosulfate titre volume is modified by the thiosulfate factor. A blank titration is not required for this assay since no heating or cooling of the reaction is involved.

Compleximetric titrations

Titrations of this type rely on the formation of complexes between metal ions and compounds capable of donating electrons to form stable, soluble complexes. Compounds of this type are called (not surprisingly) *complexing agents*, while complexing agents that form water-soluble complexes with metal ions are termed *sequestering agents*. The most commonly used agent of this sort is disodium edetate.

Disodium edetate has the structure shown in Figure 6.5 and ionises with the release of two H^+ ions. For this reason, compleximetric titrations involving disodium edetate require an alkaline pH and a buffer to ensure that the released protons do not lower the pH. The usual buffer is ammonia solution, which buffers to around pH 10. Careful choice of buffer conditions can allow the assay of several different metal ions in the same sample; for example, in the assay of Intraperitoneal Dialysis Solution BPC, both Ca^{2+} and Mg^{2+} are assayed by titration with 0.02 M disodium edetate.

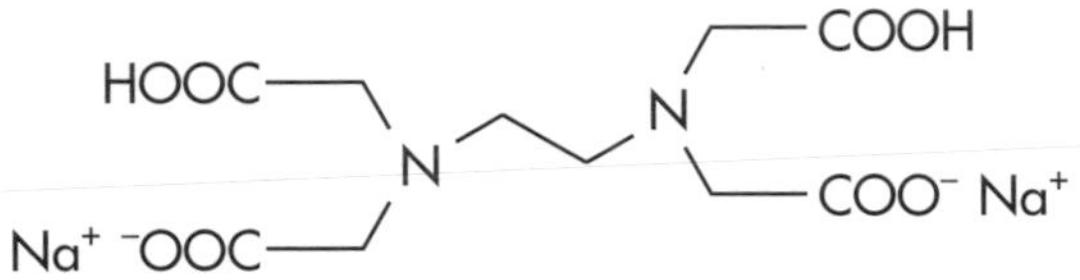

Figure 6.5 The structure of disodium edetate.

The concentration of metal ions in electrolyte preparations is often stated in millimoles per litre or sometimes millimoles per mL, where a millimole is simply one thousandth of a mole. This means that the method of deriving the equivalent relationship needs to be altered slightly from that previously stated. Using calcium ions as an example:

1 mole Ca^{2+} ions $\equiv$ 1 mole disodium edetate

1 mole Ca^{2+} ions $\equiv$ 1000 mL 1 M disodium edetate

1 millimole Ca^{2+} ions $\equiv$ 1 mL 1 M disodium edetate

0.02 millimole Ca^{2+} ions $\equiv$ 1 mL 0.02 M disodium edetate.

This implies that for every 1 mL of titrant added from the burette, 0.02 millimoles of calcium will be complexed. The relationship is called a *millimolar equivalent*.

Older readers may remember the use of milliequivalents per litre as a means of describing electrolyte concentrations. Derivation of milliequivalents relies on calculation of the *equivalent weight* of the sample.

For metal ions, the equivalent weight is found by dividing the relative atomic mass of the ion in question by its valency. In the case of monovalent ions such as Na^+ and K^+ this is straightforward, since the relative atomic mass and the equivalent weight are the same. For divalent ions such as Ca^{2+} and Mg^{2+} the equivalent weight is half the relative atomic mass, while for trivalent ions (e.g. Al^{3+}) the equivalent weight is a third of the relative atomic mass. The use of equivalent weights was discarded in pharmacy some years ago but, unfortunately, some physicians still prescribe injections and infusion solutions in terms of milliequivalents of ion per litre.

The indicators used in compleximetric titrations are usually themselves complexing agents, which form weak complexes with the metal ion when added initially. As the edetate solution is titrated, the weak complex is displaced by the stronger edetate complex to reveal the free colour of the indicator. The most commonly used indicator is known by the sinister name of *mordant black*. This indicator forms wine-red complexes with metal ions, but changes to a dark blue colour at the end point when the edetate has displaced all of the metal ions from the indicator complex.

Disodium edetate really is God's gift to undergraduates. It is a stable, water-soluble compound that gives sharp end points and, best of all, reacts with most metal ions in a 1 : 1 molar ratio irrespective of the valency of the ion. In this way, metal ions such as Zn^{2+}, Ca^{2+} and Al^{3+} can all be assayed in pharmaceutical samples.

Argentimetric titrations

As the name suggests, these assays all involve silver nitrate ($AgNO_3$). This salt is the only water-soluble salt of silver, so reaction of silver nitrate with any other salt will result in the production of a precipitate. Salts such as sodium chloride (NaCl) and potassium cyanide (KCN) can be assayed in this way.

$$AgNO_3 + NaCl \rightarrow AgCl(ppt) + NaNO_3$$
$$AgNO_3 + KCN \rightarrow AgCN(ppt) + KNO_3$$

The sample of salt is dissolved in water and titrated with standardised silver nitrate solution until all the silver salt has precipitated. Titrations of this type can be self-indicating, but usually an indicator is chosen that gives a coloured precipitate at the end point. In the assay of NaCl, potassium chromate is added to the solution; once all the NaCl has reacted, the first drop of $AgNO_3$ in excess results in the precipitation of red silver chromate, which changes the colour of the solution to one of brown-red.

Limit tests

Limit tests are quantitative or semi-quantitative tests used in the *British Pharmacopoeia* to identify and control small quantities of impurity that may be present in drug samples. A sample of the drug is reacted to produce a colour (usually) and the intensity of the colour is compared with that obtained from a known amount of standard drug. The colour obtained from the standard sample represents the absolute upper limit (hence the name of the technique) of impurity permitted in the sample of drug.

A typical example of a limit test is the test for salicylic acid in a sample of Aspirin BP. Salicylic acid is formed by hydrolysis of aspirin (or may be an impurity from the synthesis). The test involves comparing the violet colour produced when the sample is reacted with ferric chloride with that obtained from a standard salicylic acid solution.

The procedure is as follows.

> Dissolve 0.1 g of the sample in 5 mL of ethanol (96%) and add 15 mL of iced water and 0.05 mL of a 0.5% w/v solution of iron(III) chloride hexahydrate. After 1 minute the colour of the solution is not more intense than that of a solution prepared at the same time by adding a mixture of 4 mL of ethanol (96%), 0.1 mL of 5 M acetic acid, 15 mL of water and 0.05 mL of a 0.5% w/v solution of iron(III) chloride hexahydrate to 1 mL of a 0.0050% w/v solution of salicylic acid in ethanol (96%).

The absolute limit for salicylic acid in Aspirin BP is 500 ppm, as can be shown below.

1 mL of 0.0050% w/v solution of salicylic acid $\equiv$ 0.1 g aspirin

1 mL of 0.005 g/100 mL solution of salicylic acid $\equiv$ 0.1 g aspirin

1 mL of 0.00005 g/mL solution of salicylic acid $\equiv$ 0.1 g aspirin

0.00005 g salicylic acid $\equiv$ 0.1 g aspirin

50 μg salicylic acid $\equiv$ 0.1 g aspirin

500 μg salicylic acid $\equiv$ 1.0 g aspirin = 500 ppm

Problems

Q6.1 Lithium carbonate (Li_2CO_3, $M_r = 73.9$) is a drug widely used in the treatment of depression. The BP assay for lithium carbonate involves the addition of an excess of hydrochloric acid to a sample of the drug and back titration of the unreacted hydrochloric acid with sodium hydroxide.

(a) Explain why back titrations are sometimes used in volumetric analysis.

(b) Write balanced chemical equations for the reactions expressed above, and hence calculate the weight of lithium carbonate equivalent to 1 mL of 1 M HCl (the equivalent relationship).

(c) This assay was carried out and the following results were obtained

> Weight of bottle + sample = 11.7707 g
>
> Weight of bottle + residual sample = 10.7142 g
>
> Volume of 1 M ($f = 0.9989$) HCl added = 50.00 mL
>
> Burette readings, titrant 1 M ($f = 1.012$) NaOH
>
> Initial volume = 0.50 mL
>
> Final volume = 21.55 mL

(i) Calculate the percentage weight in weight of lithium carbonate in the sample.

(ii) What is the significance of an answer greater than 100%?

(iii) Suggest an indicator for this assay, and explain your reasoning.

Q6.2 Methyldopa (Figure 6.6) is a drug useful in the treatment of hypertension. The BP assay for methyldopa is as follows.

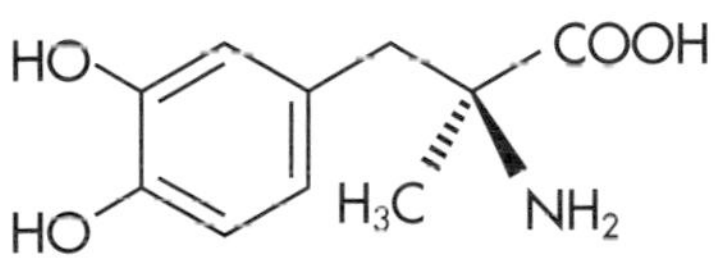

Figure 6.6 The structure of methyldopa, $M_r = 211.2$.

Weigh about 0.2 g of sample accurately and dissolve in a mixture of 15 mL of anhydrous formic acid, 30 mL of anhydrous acetic acid and 30 mL of 1,4-dioxan. Titrate with 0.1 M perchloric acid using crystal violet solution as indicator.

(a) State which technique of volumetric assay is used for methyldopa, and explain why titrations of this type are sometimes required. What precautions should be observed for assays of this type.

(b) Describe, in detail, how the perchloric acid used in this assay may be standardised (no calculation required).

(c) The above assay was carried out and the following results were obtained. Derive the equivalent relationship for this assay and hence determine the purity of the sample of methyldopa.

Weight of sample taken = 0.2016 g

Volume of 0.1 M $HClO_4$ ($f = 0.986$) required = 9.64 mL

Q6.3   Vitamin C (ascorbic acid) is used in pharmaceutical formulation as an antioxidant and also has a medical use as a vitamin. Tablets of vitamin C may be assayed by titration with complex salts of cerium. The reactions occurring are as follows and are shown in Figure 6.7.

$$\text{vitamin C} + 2Ce^{4+} \rightarrow \text{vitamin C (oxidised)} + 2Ce^{3+}$$

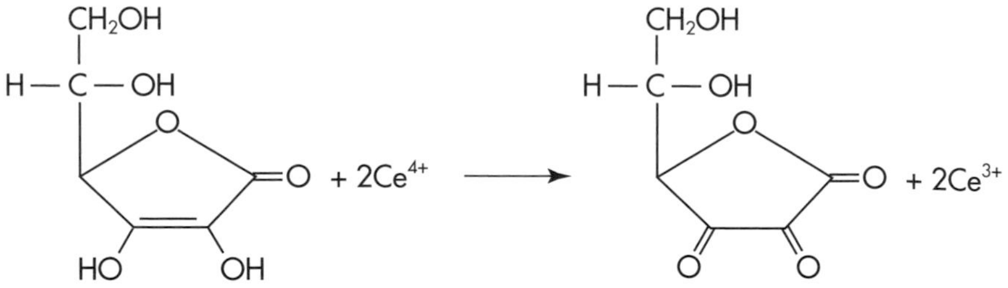

Figure 6.7   Reactions of ascorbic acid with cerium.

(a) What name is given to this type of titration?
(b) Ten 50 mg vitamin C tablets were weighed and powdered and an amount of powder equivalent to 0.15 g of

ascorbic acid was dissolved as completely as possible in a mixture of 30 mL of water and 20 mL of 1 M sulfuric acid. This sample was then titrated with 0.1 M ammonium cerium sulfate (ACS) using ferroin sulfate solution as indicator. Given that the relative molecular mass of ascorbic acid is 176.12, derive the equivalent relationship for this assay and hence calculate the percentage of the stated amount of ascorbic acid in the tablets from the following data.

Weight of 10 tablets = 6.4319 g

Weight of sample = 2.0131 g

Volume of 0.1 M ($f = 1.244$) ACS required = 15.30 mL

(c)   Ascorbic acid has pK_a values of 4.2 and 11.6. Assign the pK_a values to the structure of ascorbic acid, and explain why one acidic hydrogen is more than one million times more acidic than the other.

(Answers to problems can be found on pp. 222–224.)

7

Analytical spectroscopy

Analytical spectroscopy is the science of determining how much of a substance is present in a sample by accurately measuring how much light is absorbed or emitted by atoms or molecules within it. Different types of spectroscopy are available, depending on the type or wavelength of electromagnetic radiation absorbed or emitted by the atom or molecule. A detailed review of all types of modern instrumental analysis is beyond the scope of this book, but the use of spectroscopy in the analysis of drugs and medicines is very important and will be considered.

Light is a form of electromagnetic radiation, so called because it consists of an electric component and a magnetic component, which oscillate in mutually perpendicular directions and perpendicular to the direction of travel of the radiation through space (see Figure 7.1).

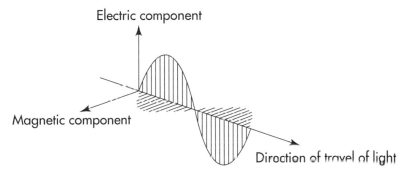

Figure 7.1 A diagram of electromagnetic radiation.

The complete spectrum of electromagnetic radiation is shown in Figure 7.2 and ranges from low-energy radio and television waves through to very high-energy gamma rays. The tiny part of the electromagnetic spectrum that human eyes can detect (approximately 400–700 nm) is called the visible spectrum, and spectroscopy carried out at these wavelengths is termed visible spectroscopy or 'colorimetry'. The part of the electromagnetic spectrum just beyond the red end of the visible spectrum is termed the *infrared* portion and has longer

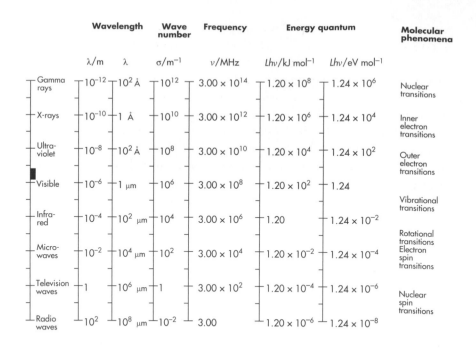

Wavelength		Wave number	Frequency	Energy quantum		Molecular phenomena
λ/m	λ	σ/m^{-1}	ν/MHz	$Lh\nu/kJ\ mol^{-1}$	$Lh\nu/eV\ mol^{-1}$	
Gamma rays 10^{-12}	10^2 Å	10^{12}	3.00×10^{14}	1.20×10^8	1.24×10^6	Nuclear transitions
X-rays 10^{-10}	1 Å	10^{10}	3.00×10^{12}	1.20×10^6	1.24×10^4	Inner electron transitions
Ultra-violet 10^{-8}	10^2 Å	10^8	3.00×10^{10}	1.20×10^4	1.24×10^2	Outer electron transitions
Visible 10^{-6}	1 μm	10^6	3.00×10^8	1.20×10^2	1.24	Vibrational transitions
Infra-red 10^{-4}	10^2 μm	10^4	3.00×10^6	1.20	1.24×10^{-2}	Rotational transitions
Micro-waves 10^{-2}	10^4 μm	10^2	3.00×10^4	1.20×10^{-2}	1.24×10^{-4}	Electron spin transitions
Television waves 1	10^6 μm	1	3.00×10^2	1.20×10^{-4}	1.24×10^{-6}	Nuclear spin transitions
Radio waves 10^2	10^8 μm	10^{-2}	3.00	1.20×10^{-6}	1.24×10^{-8}	

The visible spectrum

	Wavelength		Wave number	Energy quantum	
	λ/m		σ/m^{-1}	$Lh\nu/kJ\ mol^{-1}$	$Lh\nu/eV\ mol^{-1}$
Violet	4.00×10^{-7}		2.50×10^6	299	3.10
Blue					
Green	5.00×10^{-7}		2.00×10^6	239	2.48
Yellow	5.89×10^{-7}	(sodium D Line)			
Orange	6.00×10^{-7}		1.67×10^6	199	2.06
Red	7.00×10^{-7}		1.43×10^6	171	1.77

Figure 7.2 A diagram of the electromagnetic spectrum.

wavelength and lower energy than visible light. Similarly, the part of the spectrum beyond the violet end of the visible is called the *ultraviolet* portion and is of shorter wavelength and higher energy than visible light.

Electromagnetic radiation can be thought of as a wave-form travelling through space, and the type of radiation used in a particular experiment depends on the information required from the experiment. One feature of the radiation, which is always quoted, is the *wavelength* of the light. The wavelength is defined as the distance from one wave crest to the next (or trough to trough) and is usually quoted in nanometres (nm, 10^{-9} m) to allow for reasonably sized numbers (Figure 7.3). The symbol for wavelength is λ the Greek letter 'lambda'. The energy contained in the individual quanta of energy (photons) of a beam of radiation of a given wavelength is inversely proportional to the wavelength. This means that radio waves with wavelengths of several hundred metres have low energies, while gamma rays and X-rays are high-energy, short wavelength forms of radiation.

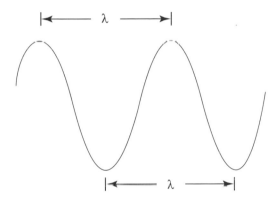

Figure 7.3 The wavelength of light.

Other terms used extensively in spectroscopy are the *wavenumber* and the *frequency*. The wavenumber is defined as the number of waves per unit of length (usually quoted in units of 'reciprocal centimetres' (cm^{-1}; where 1 cm $= 10^{-2}$ m) and is the reciprocal of the wavelength in centimetres, i.e. $1/\lambda$. The use of wavenumber is usually confined to infrared spectroscopy.

The frequency is defined as the number of waves emitted from a source per second; the unit of frequency is the hertz (Hz; 1 Hz = 1 wave per second), and the symbol for it is ν (the Greek letter 'nu').

The frequency and the wavelength are related by a constant called the speed of light, symbol c. This value (approximately 3×10^8 m s^{-1}) is the product of the frequency and the wavelength, i.e.

Velocity of light = frequency × wavelength

or

$$c = \nu \times \lambda$$

Since both frequency and wavenumber are inversely proportional to wavelength, the energy of a photon is directly proportional to both of these quantities.

When an atom or molecule is exposed to electromagnetic radiation, the energy can be absorbed in one of three ways:

1. The energy can promote an electron from a bonding orbital to a higher-energy antibonding orbital, a so-called *electronic* transition.
2. The energy can act to increase the vibration, or oscillation, of atoms about a chemical bond. This is termed a *vibrational* transition.
3. The energy can bring about an increase in the rotation of atoms about a chemical bond, which is a *rotational* transition.

In energy terms, the differences between these effects are enormous. It requires approximately 100 times more energy to bring about a vibrational transition than it does to produce a rotational one. Similarly, an electronic transition requires almost 100-fold more energy than is needed for a vibrational transition. This is important for two reasons: first, it means that each electronic transition must be associated with vibrational and rotational transitions; second, since electronic transitions require so much energy, only light of short wavelength is sufficiently energetic to bring them about. Thus, for example, infrared radiation can achieve increased vibration and rotation about chemical bonds, but has insufficient energy to promote an electron to an antibonding orbital and bring about an electronic transition. Ultraviolet or visible light is generally required to achieve electronic transitions.

Although spectroscopy can be carried out on different types of compounds, with different electronic configurations, most quantitative work (and all the examples in this book) will involve π ('pi') electron systems. The π electrons (the so-called 'mobile electrons') are the electrons found in multiple bonds. A carbon–carbon double bond contains one σ ('sigma') bond and one π bond, while a carbon–carbon triple bond consists of one σ bond and two π bonds. These π electrons are easily excited and promoted to a high-energy antibonding orbital. When the electron falls back down to the ground state, this energy is released and can be measured by a spectrophotometer.

The part of the molecule that is responsible for the absorption of light is called the *chromophore* (see Figure 7.4) and consists of a region of double or triple bonds, especially if the multiple bonds are *conjugated*, that is if the structure contains alternating multiple and single bonds. The longer the run of conjugated double or triple bonds in the molecule, the more easily the molecule will absorb light. Aromatic

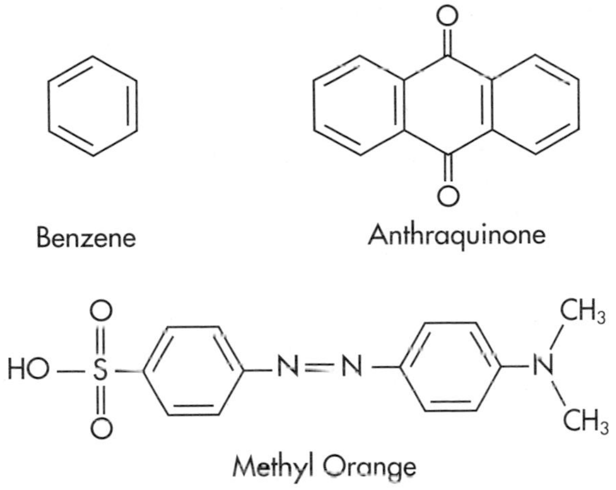

Figure 7.4 Examples of chromophores.

compounds, which contain a benzene ring, will absorb ultraviolet light of wavelength 254 nm and this property is exploited in many spectroscopic analyses and in detectors for chromatographic systems. If the chromophore is more extensive, then the molecule will be excitable by light of lower energy, until, if the chromophore is very large, visible light will have sufficient energy to excite the electrons of the chromophore and the compound will absorb visible light.

A molecule of this type, which absorbs light in the visible part of the electromagnetic spectrum, is said to be *coloured* because our eyes will detect the light reflected back from the compound, which will be the complementary colour to the light absorbed. White light, remember, is made up of all the colours of the rainbow, and can be split into its constituent colours by a prism or droplet of water. For example, if a dye molecule absorbs light of red, orange and yellow wavelengths, our eyes will detect the reflected blue, green and purple light and we will see the material as coloured blue. Similarly, a red dye will absorb the short wavelength blue light and reflect the reds and oranges back to our eyes. This property is utilised in the use of indicators for titrations (see Chapter 6) where the absorption spectrum (and hence the colour) of the indicator changes with the pH of the solution.

Effect of pH on spectra

If a graph of the extent of light absorption (measured as the quantity termed 'absorbance', defined later on p. 166) is plotted against the wavelength, then the complete absorption spectrum of a molecule can be obtained (Figure 7.5). The wavelength at which the absorbance (A) is highest is called the λ_{max} (read as 'lambda max') and is a characteristic of a particular chromophore. The λ_{max} of a compound is sometimes used in the *British Pharmacopoeia* for identification of drugs and unknown compounds.

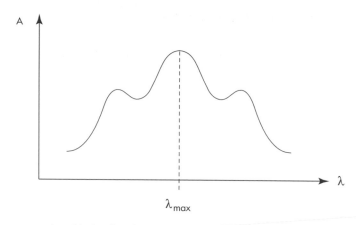

Figure 7.5 A plot of light absorbance vs λ.

The wavelength at which the λ_{max} occurs should be a constant for a given compound but, like many 'constants' in science, λ_{max} can move around and change. This is not entirely bad news, as a large amount of useful information can be obtained about a compound simply by observing any shifts that occur in λ_{max} when, for example, the compound is ionised.

A shift in λ_{max} towards longer wavelength is referred to as a *bathochromic* or red shift, because red is the colour at the long wavelength end of the visible spectrum. A bathochromic shift usually occurs due to the action of an *auxochrome*. This is a functional group attached to the chromophore which does not absorb light energy itself but which influences the wavelengths of light absorbed by the chromophore. Examples of auxochromes include the $-NH_2$, $-OH$ and $-SH$ groups. These functional groups possess lone pairs of non-bonded electrons that can interact with the π electrons of the chromophore and allow light of longer wavelength to be absorbed. A good example of this effect is to compare the λ_{max} values of benzene and aniline (also called phenylamine or aminobenzene), shown in Figure 7.6.

The λ_{max} of benzene is 204 nm, whereas the λ_{max} of aniline is 230 nm. This is due to the lone pair of electrons on the NH_2 interacting

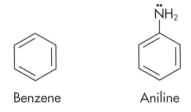

Benzene   Aniline

Figure 7.6 The structures of benzene and aniline.

with the ring electrons to increase the electron density throughout the ring, particularly at the *ortho* and *para* positions of the ring, as shown in Figure 7.7.

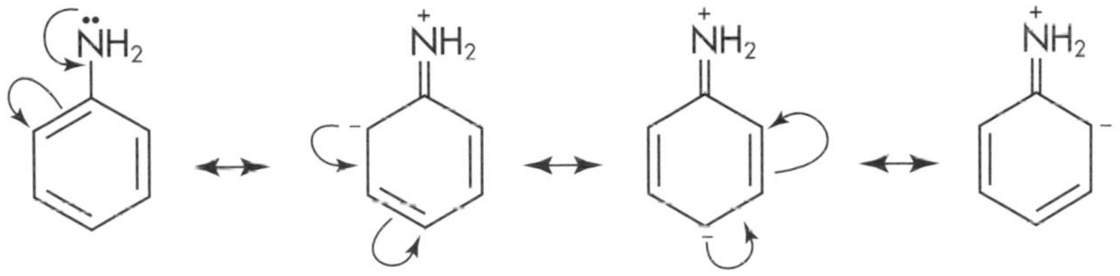

Figure 7.7 The +M effect of aniline.

This *mesomeric* (or M) effect is seen when aniline is placed in a solution of pH 8–14, i.e. when the basic aniline is unionised. When aniline is placed in a solution of pH < 7, the λ_{max} returns to virtually the value obtained for benzene (203 nm). What is happening is that aniline in acidic solution reacts to form the anilinium salt. The lone pair of electrons on the nitrogen is now involved in bond formation to an H⁺ ion and can no longer function as an auxochrome. The structure of aniline hydrochloride is shown in Figure 7.8.

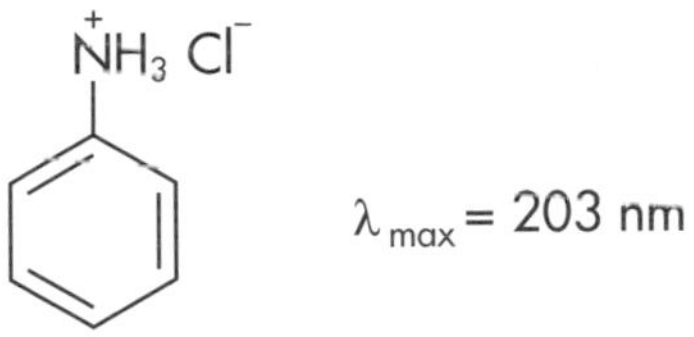

$\lambda_{max} = 203$ nm

Figure 7.8 The structure of aniline hydrochloride and its λ_{max} value.

A shift in λ_{max} to shorter wavelength is called a *hypsochromic* effect, or blue shift, and usually occurs when compounds with a basic auxochrome ionise and the lone pair is no longer able to interact with the electrons of the chromophore. Hypsochromic effects can also be seen when spectra are run in different solvents or at elevated temperatures. Spectral shifts of this type can be used to identify drugs that contain an aromatic amine functional group, e.g. the local anaesthetic benzocaine (see Figure 7.9).

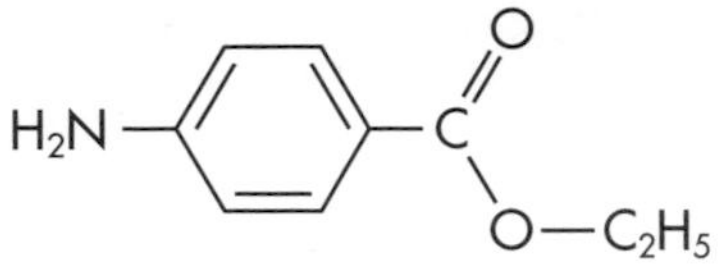

Figure 7.9 The structure of benzocaine.

Bathochromic and hypsochromic effects are seldom seen in isolation. Bathochromic effects are usually associated with increases in the intensity of light absorbed, while hypsochromic effects usually occur with decreases in absorbance. An effect that causes an increase in light absorbance is called a *hyperchromic* effect, while a decrease in the intensity of light absorbed is termed a *hypochromic* effect. The four words used to describe shifts in λ_{max} could almost have been chosen to cause maximum confusion among students trying to remember the terms. Perhaps the best way to remember the terms is to say that hyper- means an increase, hypo- a decrease, and that a shift to longer wavelength is a red shift while a shift to shorter wavelength is a blue shift, or, alternatively, commit to memory Figure 7.10. Hyperchromic effects are used in anticancer drug research to measure the extent of drug binding to DNA. If a solution of duplex, or double-stranded, DNA is gently heated, the double helix will start to unwind, exposing the heterocyclic bases in the centre of the duplex. This can be observed experimentally as the absorbance of the DNA solution at 260 nm will increase, causing a hyperchromic effect. Drugs that bind to DNA stabilise the molecule and reduce the extent of the observed hyperchromicity.

Drugs that contain phenolic groups, e.g. paracetamol (see Figure 7.11), also show spectral shifts on ionisation. In the case of phenols, which are weak acids with a pK_a of approximately 10, ionisation increases the intensity of light absorption and the position of λ_{max} moves to longer wavelength. This is because ionisation and loss of the H atom as an H^+ ion results in a full negative charge on the oxygen (a phenoxide ion), which can interact with the ring more effectively than the lone pair of electrons present in the unionised molecule. This is shown for phenol in Figure 7.11.

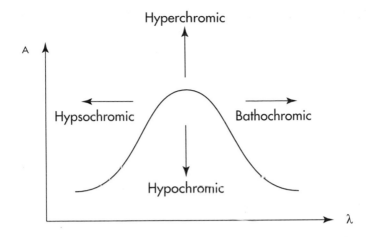

Figure 7.10   Changes that occur in λ_{max}.

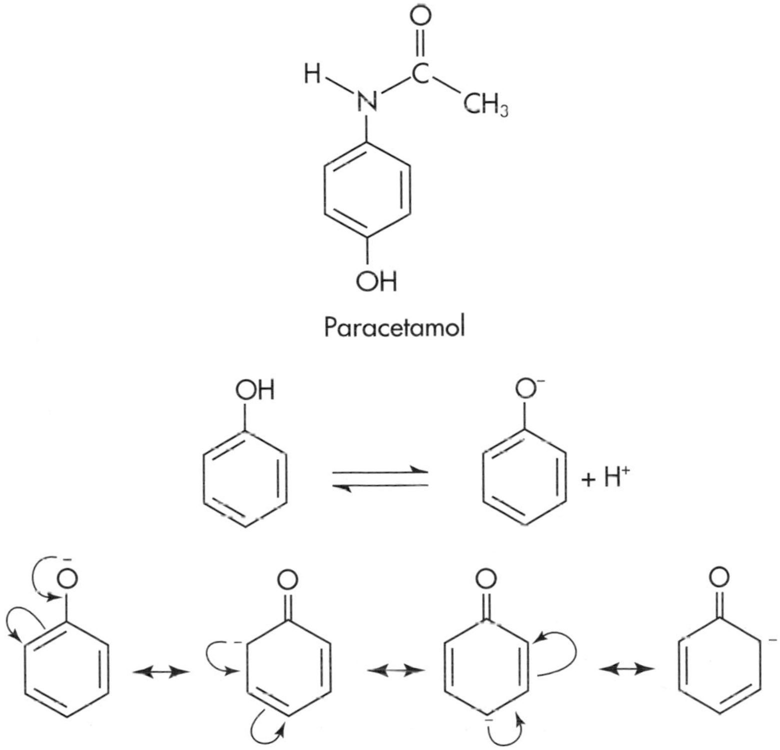

Paracetamol

Figure 7.11   The structure of paracetamol and ionisation of phenols.

Instrumentation

An instrument that measures the intensity of light absorbed by atoms or molecules is called a *spectrophotometer*. Different types of spectrophotometers exist depending on whether they use a single beam of light or separate reference and sample beams, and on whether they measure at a fixed wavelength or scan the absorption spectrum at many wavelengths. As with most analytical instruments, accuracy, precision and cost vary widely.

In general, all spectrophotometers have a layout similar to the one shown in Figure 7.12.

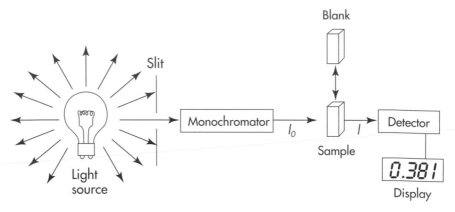

Figure 7.12   A schematic diagram of a spectrophotometer.

Light source

The source or lamp is really two separate lamps which, taken together, cover the whole of the visible and ultraviolet regions of the electromagnetic spectrum. For white visible light a *tungsten* lamp is used. This lamp is nothing more sophisticated than a light bulb with a filament made of the metal tungsten. You are probably reading this book by the light of one of these lamps. A tungsten lamp emits light of wavelengths 350–2000 nm and is adequate for colorimetry.

For compounds that absorb in the ultraviolet region of the spectrum, a *deuterium* lamp is required. Deuterium is one of the heavy isotopes of hydrogen, possessing one neutron more than ordinary hydrogen in its nucleus. A deuterium lamp is a high-energy source that emits light of approximately 200–370 nm and is used for all spectroscopy in the ultraviolet region of the spectrum.

Fixed-wavelength instruments allow the operator to select which lamp is required for an assay, whereas scanning instruments, which produce a plot of the whole absorption spectrum of the sample, switch lamps automatically.

Monochromator

For most quantitative measurements light must be *monochromatic*, i.e. of one particular wavelength. This is achieved by passing the polychromatic light (i.e. light of many wavelengths) through a monochromator. There are two types of monochromator in modern spectrophotometers: *prisms* or *diffraction gratings*.

A prism is a triangular piece of quartz that refracts (or bends) light passing through it. The extent of the refraction depends on the wavelength of the light, so a beam of white light can be split into its component colours by passage through a prism. The prism is then rotated to select a particular wavelength required for the assay (Figure 7.13). This effect is identical to the formation of a rainbow when light from the sun is split into its seven component colours (red, orange, yellow, green, blue, indigo and violet) by refraction through droplets of rain.

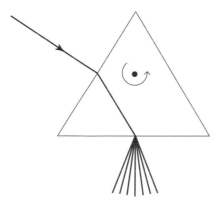

Figure 7.13 A diagram of a prism.

A diffraction grating is a small piece of mirrored glass onto which a large number of equally spaced lines have been cut, several thousand per millimetre of grating, to give a structure that looks like a small comb. The spaces between the cuts are approximately equal to the wavelengths of light and so a beam of polychromatic light will be refracted into its component wavelengths by the grating. The grating is then rotated to select the wavelength desired for assay (Figure 7.14).

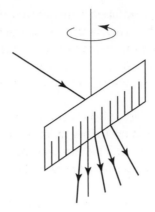

Figure 7.14 A diagram of a diffraction grating.

Detector

After light has passed through the sample, any decrease in intensity, due to absorption, is measured by a detector. This is usually a clever piece of electronics called a *photomultiplier tube* (see Figure 7.15), which acts to convert the intensity of the beam of light into an electrical signal that can be measured easily, and then also acts as an amplifier to increase the

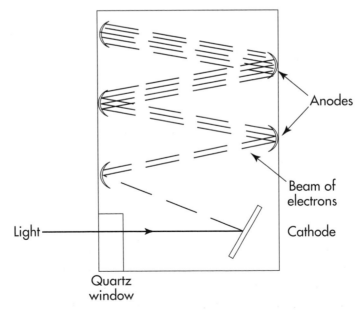

Figure 7.15 A diagram of a photomultiplier tube.

strength of the signal still further. Light enters the tube and strikes the cathode; this releases electrons, which are attracted to an anode above. When the electrons strike this anode they release more electrons, which are, in turn, attracted to the anode above that, where the process is repeated. In this way a cascade of electrons is generated and the signal is amplified.

Once the electrical signal leaves the photomultiplier tube, it is fed to a recorder if a printout is required, or, more usually, to a screen where the absorption spectrum can be displayed. Most modern spectrophotometers are now interfaced to a personal computer to allow storage of large amounts of data, or to allow access to a library of stored spectra on the hard drive of the machine. This allows comparison of stored spectra with the experimentally derived results from the laboratory and aids in the identification of unknown compounds.

Experimental measurement of absorbance

The sequence of events in making a measurement with a spectrophotometer is as follows.

1. The monochromator is set to the wavelength of measurement, the shutter is closed to prevent light reaching the detector, and the instrument is set to infinite absorbance. This is often done automatically during the 'warm-up' by modern instruments.
2. The shutter is opened, the solvent (or 'blank') is placed in the light path and the instrument is set to zero absorbance. The blank is usually just the solvent for the assay but, strictly speaking, should be everything in the sample matrix except the sample being measured. This means that in complex assays the blank solution has to be made up to match exactly the composition of the solvent/medium in which the sample will be measured, and has to be extracted or otherwise treated in exactly the same way as the sample.
3. The sample solution (or 'test') is placed in the light path and the absorbance is read directly by the instrument.

Dilutions

The most important part of any spectroscopic assay is not the performance of the spectrophotometer (although the accuracy of the instrument is checked periodically). The crucial part of any experiment is the accurate preparation of the test and standard solutions. This often involves the accurate dilution of a stock solution using the volumetric glassware introduced in Chapter 6, namely the pipette and the volumetric flask.

A common procedure is to prepare a range of dilutions for use as a calibration graph as in the worked example below.

Worked example

You are presented with a stock solution containing a $50\,\mu\mathrm{g\,mL^{-1}}$ solution of a drug. Prepare 100 mL of solution to contain 5, 10, 20 and $30\,\mu\mathrm{g\,mL^{-1}}$ of drug.

The first step is to calculate how much of the $50\,\mu\mathrm{g\,mL^{-1}}$ stock solution will be required for each dilution. This can be done by using the relationship below

$$\frac{[\text{Required}]}{[\text{Stock}]} \times \text{volume required}$$

where [ ] represent the concentrations of drug. This relationship may be more easily remembered as

$$\frac{[\text{Want}]}{[\text{Got}]} \times \text{volume of flask}$$

Using this relationship, the $30\,\mu\mathrm{g\,mL^{-1}}$ solution is prepared from $(30/50) \times 100 = 60$ mL of stock solution made up to 100 mL with solvent. The $20\,\mu\mathrm{g\,mL^{-1}}$ solution is prepared from $(20/50) \times 100 = 40$ mL of stock made up to 100 mL with solvent, and so on for all the dilutions.

The alternative way to prepare these dilutions is to prepare each dilution from the next most concentrated. This is called a *serial dilution* and is carried out as follows. The $30\,\mu\mathrm{g\,mL^{-1}}$ and $20\,\mu\mathrm{g\,mL^{-1}}$ solutions are prepared as above. The $10\,\mu\mathrm{g\,mL^{-1}}$ solution is prepared from the $20\,\mu\mathrm{g\,mL^{-1}}$ solution (50 mL of $20\,\mu\mathrm{g\,mL^{-1}}$ solution made up to 100 mL with solvent) and the $5\,\mu\mathrm{g\,mL^{-1}}$ solution is prepared from the $10\,\mu\mathrm{g\,mL^{-1}}$ solution in the same way. A serial dilution has the advantage of using less of the stock solution (100 mL compared to 130 mL in this example) and is used whenever the drug or reagent in question is expensive or in short supply.

Quantitative aspects of spectroscopy

Light passing through a substance decreases in intensity as a result of three processes:

1.   Reflection at phase boundaries (liquid/air, glass/liquid, etc.). This is caused by differences in the refractive index of the different materials through which the light is passing.

2.   Scattering of light caused by non-homogeneity of the sample.
3.   Absorbance by atoms or molecules in solution.

Loss of intensity due to point (1) can be compensated by use of an appropriate blank solution since phase boundary effects should be the same in the test and blank solutions.

The scattering effects in point (2) can be minimised by careful sample preparation, i.e. ensuring the sample dissolves completely in the chosen solvent, that there are no air bubbles adhering to the sample cell, and that there are no fingerprints, dust, mascara, dandruff or other unwanted material on the outside of the cell which will affect the accuracy of the absorbance measurements.

Losses in intensity due to point (3) are what we are interested in measuring.

Beer's and Lambert's laws

The quantitative aspects of spectrophotometry are based on two very similar laws. The first is Beer's law (Figure 7.16), which states that 'the intensity of a beam of parallel, monochromatic light decreases exponentially with the concentration of the absorbing molecules'. Beer's law can be expressed mathematically as

$$I = I_0 e^{-k'c} \tag{7.1}$$

where I_0 is intensity of light incident on the sample, I is intensity of light transmitted by the sample, k' is a constant and c is the concentration of the sample.

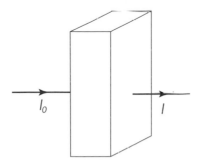

Figure 7.16 A diagram of Beer's law.

Taking logarithms,

$$\log \frac{I_0}{I} = k'c$$

Log (I_0/I) is a dimensionless quantity (strictly speaking a logarithm of a ratio of light intensities) and is defined as *absorbance*. Absorbance is the quantity measued and plotted in spectrophotometry.

Thus Beer's law states that absorbance is proportional to concentration.

The second relationship is Lambert's law, which states that the 'intensity of a beam of parallel, monochromatic light decreases exponentially as the light travels through a thickness of homogeneous medium', expresses mathematically as

$$I = I_0 e^{-k''l} \tag{7.2}$$

where I and I_0 are as before, l is thickness of the medium (or path length) through which the light passes and k'' is (another) constant.

Taking logarithms,

$$\log \frac{I_0}{I} = k''l$$

i.e. absorbance is proportional to path length.

These two fundamental equations are so similar that they can be combined into one relationship, the Beer–Lambert law or equation, which can be expressed as

$$\textbf{Absorbance} = \log \frac{I_0}{I} = \textbf{\textit{kcl}} \tag{7.3}$$

Here k is yet another constant, the value of which depends on the units used for the concentration, c.

If the units of concentration are molarity (i.e. number of moles per litre), then the constant is ε (the Greek letter 'epsilon') and is known as the *molar absorbtivity*. ε has units of L mol^{-1} cm^{-1}, although the units are seldom expressed. ε is equal to the absorbance of a 1 M solution in a cell of path length 1 cm and is usually a large number, approximately 10 000–20 000. In this case the Beer–Lambert equation is written as

$$A = \varepsilon c l \tag{7.4}$$

When the concentration of the sample is expressed in percentage weight in volume (% w/v) (i.e. g/100 mL) the constant used is A 1%, 1 cm, usually written as A_1^1, and is called the *specific absorbance*, with units of dL g^{-1} cm^{-1} although, again, the A_1^1 value is usually quoted without units. The A_1^1 value is very useful in pharmacy and pharmaceutical analyses where the molecular weight of the sample may be unknown (e.g. when analysing a macromolecule, such as a protein) or where a mixture of several components is being analysed in the same sample. This gives the most useful form of the Beer–Lambert equation:

$$A = A_1^1 cl \qquad (7.5)$$

It follows from the derivations above that ε and A_1^1 are related, and either one can be calculated from the other by using equation (7.6):

$$\varepsilon = \frac{A_1^1 \times \text{relative molecular mass}}{10} \qquad (7.6)$$

As mentioned above, absorbance is defined as log I_0/I; older textbooks refer to the term as *extinction*, while even older manuscripts call it *optical density*. All three terms mean the same, but 'absorbance' is the expression that should be used in all analytical spectroscopy.

Two other expressions of light intensity occur in spectroscopy:

- *Transmittance*, defined as the ratio I/I_0
- *Percentage transmittance*, which is the same ratio expressed as a percentage, i.e. $100I/I_0$

The use of these two terms in analytical spectroscopy is limited to infrared spectroscopy since neither term, unlike absorbance, gives a linear relationship if plotted against concentration.

Methods of drug assay

There are two methods of using spectroscopic measurements in drug analysis, the *absolute* and the *comparative* methods of assay, and the one used depends on which side of the Atlantic Ocean you carry out the analysis.

In the UK and Europe the Beer–Lambert equation tends to be used in what is called the absolute method of assay. In this procedure the absorbance is measured experimentally and the Beer–Lambert equation is solved for c, the drug concentration. For this reason, the *British Pharmacopoeia* and *European pharmacopoeia* quote A_1^1 values in drug monographs.

In the *US Pharmacopoeia*, the comparative method of assay is preferred. In this type of assay a standard solution of the drug to be analysed is prepared, the absorbances of the sample and the standard are measured under identical conditions, and the concentration of the sample is calculated from the relationship

$$\frac{A_{\text{test}}}{A_{\text{std}}} = \frac{[\text{test}]}{[\text{std}]} \qquad (7.7)$$

where [test] is the concentration of the sample and [std] is the concentration of the prepared standard. The comparative method of assay has the advantage that it can be used even if the drug undergoes a chemical reaction during the assay (e.g. formation of a coloured derivative to allow measurement in the visible region of the spectrum), but suffers from the disadvantage that an authentic sample of the drug in question must be available for comparison.

When carrying out drug assays by spectroscopy it is often necessary to prepare a range of concentrations of a standard sample of the analyte and measure the absorbance of each solution. When these data are plotted, a straight line of positive slope should be obtained that passes through the origin. Constructing graphs of this type not only confirms that the Beer–Lambert law applies to the assay at the wavelength of measurement but also allows the graph to be used for calibration purposes. A solution of unknown concentration is prepared in exactly the same way as the standards and its absorbance is measured at the same wavelength as the standards. This absorbance is then read off the calibration graph and the concentration is calculated. Standard solutions prepared separately from the sample in this way are known as *external standards*.

A more rigorous technique involves the use of *internal standards*. An internal standard is a compound that is similar in chemical structure and physical properties to the sample being analysed. The internal standard should be added to the sample in question before extraction or assay commences and is then present in the sample matrix throughout the subsequent assay. In the assay of complex samples, some sample pretreatment is usually required and the recovery of the sample from the extraction process may not be 100%. If an internal standard is used, losses in sample will be mirrored by similar losses in the standard and the ratio of sample to standard should remain constant. Internal standards are particularly used in chromatographic analysis (especially gas chromatography and high-performance liquid chromatography), where fluctuations in instrumental parameters (e.g. flow rate of mobile phase) affect accuracy.

In certain spectroscopic analyses a similar approach to the use of internal standards is employed. This is the technique of *standard additions*. This involves addition of increasing volumes of a standard solution of the analyte to a fixed volume of the sample and construction of a calibration graph. The graph in a standard addition assay is of positive slope but intersects the y-axis at a positive value of absorbance. The amount of drug in the sample is found by extrapolation of the calibration graph back to the point where the line intersects the x-axis (i.e. when $y = 0$ in the equation of the line) as shown in Figure 7.17.

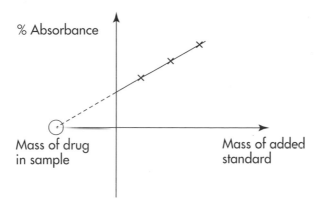

Figure 7.17   A calibration graph using method of standard additions.

The method of standard additions is widely used in atomic spectroscopy (e.g. determination of Ca^{2+} ions in serum by atomic emission spectrophotometry) and, since several aliquots of sample are analysed to produce the calibration graph, should increase the accuracy and precision of the assay.

Infrared spectroscopy

Infrared (IR) spectroscopy is a very useful technique for the identification of unknown compounds, e.g. products from a synthesis or urinary metabolites from an animal experiment, especially when used in conjunction with other structure elucidation techniques such as nuclear magnetic resonance and mass spectrometry.

The infrared region of the electromagnetic spectrum refers to light of wavelength 2.5–to 15 μm (i.e. 2.5×10^{-6} to 15×10^{-6} m) and the absorption of this light by the molecule causes changes in the vibrational energy of the molecule in its ground state. As stated previously, vibrational transitions are always associated with changes in the rotation of atoms about chemical bonds. This is analogous to electronic transitions in the absorption of ultraviolet energy, which also result in vibrational and rotational transitions. The usefulness of IR stems from the fact that each peak on the spectrum can be assigned to a particular bond, or functional group in the molecule. This often means that IR spectra are complex, with perhaps as many as 20 or 30 peaks on one spectrum.

Identification of chemical unknowns is made easier, however, because certain functional groups always appear in the same region of the IR spectrum.

Single bonds (e.g. O—H, N—H, C—H) absorb in the high-frequency part of the spectrum (approximately 4000–2100 cm^{-1}). This is because the low mass of the hydrogen atom allows vibrations to occur at high frequency. Triple bonds (e.g. in CN$^-$) absorb at approximately 2100–1900 cm^{-1}, while double bonds (e.g. C=O, C=C) absorb at approximately 1900–1500 cm^{-1}. The region of the IR spectrum corresponding to wavenumber less than approximately 1500 cm^{-1} is due to stretching of the molecule as a whole and the peaks in this region are more difficult to assign accurately. This region of the spectrum is called the *fingerprint region*, since the pattern of peaks occurring in this region is characteristic of the compound in question *and no other*. Use is made of this property in the *British Pharmacopoeia* where two samples are said to be identical when the IR spectra, obtained under identical conditions, coincide completely – i.e. the same peaks are present in the same positions with the same intensities. Reference IR spectra of authentic samples of a drug are published in the BP to verify the identity of unknown samples.

Quantitative analysis using infrared spectroscopy

The Beer–Lambert rules derived above (equation 7.3) apply equally to absorbance of infrared radiation by molecules. Moreover, infrared absorption spectra possess an advantage over the more common ultraviolet absorption in the greater number of bands present. It is often possible to select an absorption band for each component of a mixture such that little or no interference occurs between them. For these reasons, infrared spectroscopy is often used quantitatively in the analytical laboratory to determine drug concentrations in solution. A calibration curve for the assay may be obtained (and Beer's law confirmed) by converting the printed spectrum into I_0 and I using the *baseline technique* as shown in Figure 7.18. The distance from the baseline to the bottom of the page is designated I_0, the light available for absorption, while the distance from the apex of the peak to the bottom of the page is designated I, the light transmitted through the sample. The logarithm (to base 10) of the ratio I_0/I is obtained as before to yield absorbance. Note that infrared spectra are usually plotted 'upside down' so that zero absorbance is at the top of the spectrum (as usually displayed) and 100% absorbance is

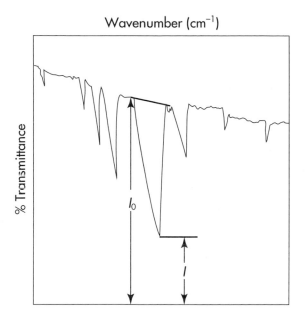

Figure 7.18 The application of the baseline technique.

at the bottom. Note also, that infrared spectroscopy is idiosyncratic in using wavenumber ('reciprocal centimetres', cm^{-1}) instead of wavelength along the x-axis and percentage transmittance instead of absorbance on the y-axis.

A major difference between infrared and ultraviolet spectroscopy is in the concentrations required for assay. In infrared spectroscopy as much as a 10% w/v solution of sample must be prepared. This means that the path length of the cells used in infrared must be very short, usually 0.025–0.1 mm (otherwise absorbance values would be too high). Another problem with infrared spectra is that the solvent used in the assay (usually chloroform or dichloromethane) also possesses chemical bonds and will absorb infrared radiation in some part of the spectrum, obscuring the absorption by the sample at these wavelengths. Samples are prepared in solution, in a mull or paste made with liquid paraffin (Nujol), or in a solid disc prepared by trituration with dry potassium bromide followed by compression in a hydraulic press.

Fluorimetry

Fluorimetry is an analytical technique that relies on the emission of electromagnetic energy by molecules. The chromophore of the molecule must be capable of absorbing light (usually in the ultraviolet region of the electromagnetic spectrum) and emitting it again (usually in the visible portion of the spectrum) to be measured by a detector. To do this, the chromophore (sometimes called the *fluorophore*) must be shielded from the normal processes that account for energy loss in the excited state (e.g. collision between molecules). The light that is emitted by the sample *is always of longer wavelength (i.e. lower energy) than the light absorbed by the molecule.* This is because the energy transfer process occurring within the excited state of the molecule is not 100% efficient. Some of the absorbing energy is lost (e.g. in vibrational transitions) and so the light emitted as fluorescence is of lower energy than the light absorbed.

The instruments used to measure fluorescence, spectrofluorimeters, require a high-energy light source (usually a xenon arc lamp) to deliver the energy required to excite the molecule, and the detector of the instrument is usually aligned at 90° to the source to minimise detection of light directly from the light source. A spectrofluorimeter also requires two monochromators, one to select the wavelength of excitation light and the other to select the wavelength of light emitted by the sample. Analytical spectrofluorimetry is widely used in pharmaceutical analysis, particularly for the assay of highly potent drugs present in medicines in tiny amounts.

There are two main advantages in the use of fluorimetry over ultraviolet spectroscopy:

1. The presence of two monochromators, and the fact that not all molecules with a chromophore fluoresce, means that fluorimetry is more specific than ordinary ultraviolet spectroscopy. This allows drugs that fluoresce to be assayed in the presence of other compounds that would interfere in an ultraviolet assay.
2. Fluorimetry is approximately 100 times more sensitive than ultraviolet spectroscopy and is ideal for the analysis of very small amounts of potent drugs. Examples are the steroids digoxin in Digoxin Tablets BP and the contraceptive agent ethinylestradiol, which is present at levels of only 30 μg per tablet.

Quenching

This phenomenon, as its name suggests, is a reduction in the intensity of light emitted during fluorescence. There are two types: self-quenching and quenching by other, non-fluorescent agents.

Self-quenching is seen at high sample concentrations (e.g. approximately 0.005% w/v) and is due to fluorescence concentrating at the irradiated face of the sample cell, instead of distributing throughout the cell. A plot of intensity of light emitted versus concentration should be linear (obeying the Beer–Lambert law). If the linearity of the graph falls off at high concentration, self-quenching should be suspected. If self-quenching of fluorescence is a problem during an assay, dilution of the sample (e.g. to 0.000 05% w/v) should eliminate the problem and restore linearity.

Quenching of fluorescence also occurs due to the action of other, non-fluorescent compounds. The most common quenching agents encountered in pharmaceutical analysis are halide ions (Cl^-, Br^-, I^-). The fluorescence of a drug such as quinine is much lower if the sample is dissolved in hydrochloric acid than it is if the quinine is dissolved in sulfuric acid, even though the concentrations of the quinine and the pH of the solutions are kept constant. Quinine is an interesting compound (Figure 7.19). It is an alkaloid extracted from the bark of the *Cinchona* tree and was used extensively for the treatment of malaria. It is a very bitter substance and is responsible for the characteristic bitter taste of tonic water. An acidic solution of quinine displays a deep blue fluorescence, which can often be observed in the glass of someone drinking tonic water (with or without gin) in a bar or club with ultraviolet lights.

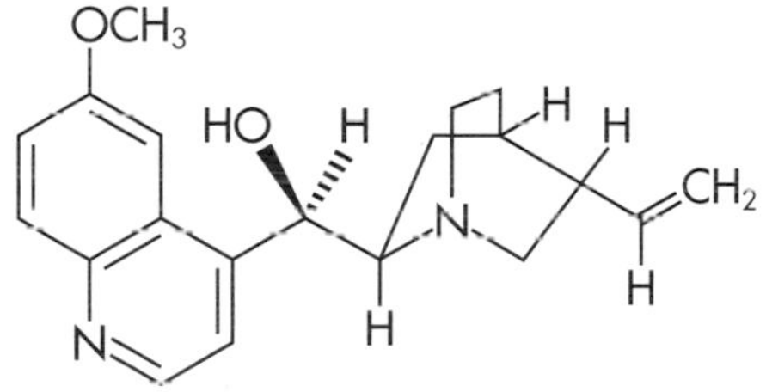

Figure 7.19 The structure of quinine.

Tutorial examples

1 *Five standard solutions of a drug (relative molecular mass 288.4) were prepared in spectroscopy-grade ethanol and the absorbance of each solution was measured at 285 nm in 1 cm cells*

Concentration (mg/100 mL)	Absorbance
1.25	0.697
1.00	0.562
0.75	0.421
0.50	0.281
0.25	0.140

(a)   Is Beer's law obeyed for this drug at this wavelength?
(b)   Calculate the A_1^1 and molar absorptivity for this drug at 285 nm.
(c)   Calculate the % transmittance given by a 0.5 mg/100 mL solution in a 2 cm cell.

1(a) Whenever a column of numbers appears in an examination question it is crying out for a graph to be plotted. In this case a plot of absorbance versus concentration yields a straight line through the origin and confirms Beer's law for this drug at this (and only this) wavelength.

(b)   The A_1^1 value is simply determined from the gradient of the graph obtained in (a) if the units of concentration are converted to percentage weight in volume. The path length of the cell is 1 cm, so the Beer–Lambert equation simplifies to a $y = mx$ type of equation with the slope $= A_1^1$.

Alternatively, the A_1^1 value can be obtained by calculation.

$$1 \text{ mg/100 mL} = 0.001 \text{ g/100 mL}$$
$$= 0.001\% \text{ w/v}$$
$$A = A_1^1 cl$$

Hence,

$$0.562 = A_1^1 \times 0.001 \times 1$$

Therefore,

$$A_1^1 = 562$$

In practice, A_1^1 would be calculated for each solution and the answers averaged.

The molar absorptivity, ε can be calculated as follows.

$$\frac{1 \text{ mg}}{100 \text{ mL}} = 0.01 \text{ g L}^{-1}$$

$$= \frac{0.01}{288.4 \text{ mol L}^{-1}}$$

$$A = \varepsilon c l$$

Hence,

$$0.562 = \varepsilon \times \frac{0.01}{288.4} \times 1$$

Therefore,

$$\varepsilon = 16\ 210$$

Note that ε, the absorbance of a 1 molar solution, is much greater than A_1^1, the absorbance of a 1% w/v solution.

(c)   The first step to calculating the percentage transmittance is to calculate the absorbance of the 0.5 mg/100 mL solution. Using A_1^1 and converting the units of concentration to percentage weight in volume,

$$A = 562 \times 0.0005 \times 2$$
$$A = 0.562$$

Unsurprisingly, this is the same absorbance as given by twice the concentration measured in a cell of half the thickness. Hence,

$$\log \frac{I_0}{I} = 0.562$$

Therefore,

$$\frac{I_0}{I} = 3.648$$

and

$$\% \text{ Transmittance} = 100 \frac{I}{I_0} = 100 \times \frac{1}{3.648} = 27.4\%$$

i.e. for this solution, 72.6% of available light is absorbed and 27.4% is transmitted.

Q 2 *The A_1^1 of cocaine at its λ_{max} is 430. In an experiment, 11.2 mg of cocaine was weighed and made up to 1 litre with 0.1 M HCl. If the measured absorbance in a 1 cm quartz cell was 0.470, calculate the purity of the sample of cocaine.*

A 2 The first step is to solve the Beer–Lambert equation:

$$A = A_1^1 cl$$
$$= 430 \times c \times 1$$

Therefore,

$$c = \frac{0.470}{430} = 0.001093\% \text{ w/v}$$

Note that if A_1^1 is used, the units of concentration must be percentage weight in volume, i.e. g/100 mL:

$$0.001093 \text{ g/100 mL}^{-1} = 10.93 \text{ mg L}^{-1}$$

However, 11.20 mg were weighed and, therefore,

$$\% \text{ Purity of sample} = \frac{10.93}{11.20} \times 100 = 97.6\%$$

Problems

Q7.1 The assay for Diazepam Tablets BP is as follows.

Weigh and powder 20 tablets. To a quantity of the powder containing 10 mg of diazepam, add 5 mL of water, mix and allow to stand for 15 minutes. Add 70 mL of a 0.5% w/v solution of sulfuric acid in methanol, shake for 15 minutes, add sufficient of the methanolic sulfuric acid to produce 100 mL and filter.

Dilute 10 mL of the filtrate to 50 mL with the same solvent and measure the absorbance of the resulting solution at the maximum at 248 nm. Calculate the content of $C_{16}H_{13}ClN_2O$ taking 450 as the value of A_1^1 at this wavelength.

(a) Draw the part of the molecule responsible for the absorption of light in this assay (see Figure 7.20). What is this part of the molecule called?

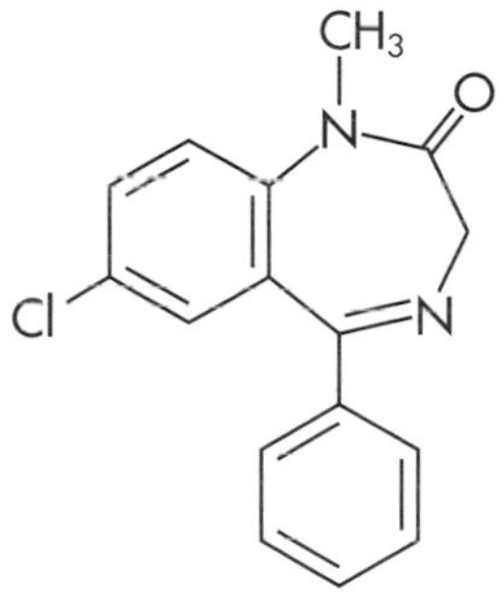

Figure 7.20 The structure of diazepam.

(b) What assumptions are made in this assay?
(c) When this assay was carried out on 5 mg diazepam tablets, the following results were obtained:

> Weight of 20 tablets = 7.4878 g
>
> Weight of sample taken = 0.7450 g
>
> Absorbance of a 1 cm layer at 284 nm = 0.848

Calculate the content of diazepam in a tablet of average weight and hence calculate the percentage of the stated amount of diazepam in the tablets.

(d) Suggest another assay method for the determination of diazepam in Diazepam Tablets.

Q7.2 Mepyramine (Figure 7.21) is an antihistamine used in the treatment of insect bites and stings. The BP assay for 50 mg Mepyramine Tablets is as follows.

Weigh and powder 20 tablets. To a quantity of the powder containing 0.1 g of mepyramine, add 75 mL of water and 5 mL of 2 M hydrochloric acid, shake vigorously for 15 minutes and dilute to 100 mL with water. To 10 mL of this solution add 10 mL of 0.1 M hydrochloric acid, centrifuge and dilute to 100 mL with water. Measure the absorbance of the resulting solution at the maximum at 316 nm taking 206 as the value of A_1^1.

This assay was carried out and the following data were obtained.

Weight of 20 tablets = 2.1361 g

Weight of sample used in assay = 0.2214 g

Absorbance at 316 nm (measured in 1 cm cell) = 0.225

(a) Calculate the content of mepyramine in a tablet of average weight and the % stated amount.

(b) Why was the sample centrifuged prior to assay?

(c) Using the structure shown in Figure 7.21 as a guide, classify mepyramine as acidic, basic or neutral and hence explain the role of the hydrochloric acid in this assay.

(d) Explain fully how the blank solution for this assay would be prepared.

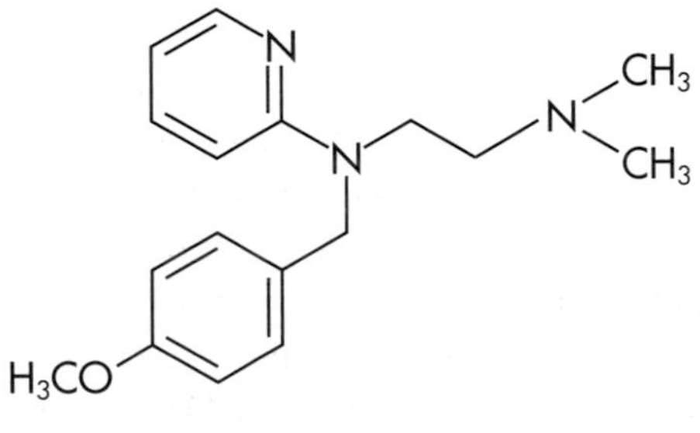

Figure 7.21 The structure of mepyramine.

(Answers to problems can be found on p. 224.)

8

Stability of drugs and medicines

Drugs sometimes have quite complicated chemical structures and are, by definition, biologically active compounds. It should not, therefore, come as a surprise that these reactive molecules undergo chemical reactions that result in their decomposition and deterioration, and that these processes begin as soon as the drug is synthesised or the medicine is formulated. Decomposition reactions of this type lead to, at best, drugs and medicines that are less active than intended (i.e. of low *efficacy*); in the worst-case scenario, decomposition can lead to drugs that are actually toxic to the patient. This is clearly bad news to all except lawyers, so the processes of decomposition and deterioration must be understood in order to minimise the risk to patients.

There are almost as many ways in which drugs can decompose as there are drugs in the *British Pharmacopoeia*, but most instability can be accounted for by the processes of *oxidation* and *hydrolysis*.

Oxidation

Oxidation is the process whereby an atom increases the number of bonds it has to oxygen, decreases the number of bonds it has to hydrogen, or loses electrons. The deterioration of drugs by oxidation requires the presence of molecular oxygen and proceeds under mild conditions. Elemental molecular oxygen, or O_2, possesses a diradical (unpaired triplet) electronic configuration in the ground state and is said to be *paramagnetic* (a species with all its electrons paired is called *diagmagnetic*). The structure of oxygen can be represented as $\cdot O{=}O\cdot$ or $O{=}O$ depending on whether the molecular orbital or valence bond theory is employed. The important fact for drug stability is that the radical species possesses two unpaired electrons, which can initiate chain reactions resulting in the breakdown of drug molecules, particularly if the reaction occurs in the presence of catalysts such as light, heat, some metal ions and peroxides. The types of drugs that are affected include phenols (such as morphine), catecholamines (for example, adrenaline (epinephrine) and noradrenaline (norepinephrine)) as well as polyunsaturated compounds such as oils, fats and fat-soluble vitamins (e.g. vitamins A and E). Radical chain reactions of this type are called *autoxidation* reactions and can be quite complicated. All, however, proceed via a number of discrete steps, namely, *initiation*, *propagation* and *termination*.

Initiation

Initiation involves homolytic fission of a covalent bond in the drug molecule to produce free radicals (Figure 8.1). The energy source for this process often comes from light, either ultraviolet or visible, falling onto the sample. Light of these wavelengths is sufficiently energetic to bring about cleavage of the pair of electrons in a covalent bond to yield two radicals.

Stage 1   Chain initiation: involves homolytic fission to produce free radicals.

$$\text{Drug} : \text{H} \longrightarrow \text{Drug}^{\bullet} + \text{H}^{\bullet}$$

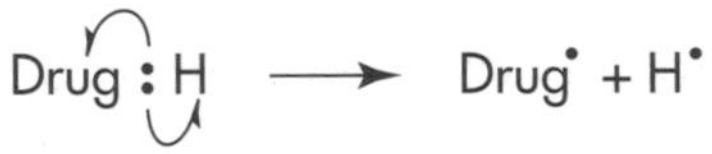

Figure 8.1   The mechanism of initiation.

Propagation

Propagation is the main part of the chemical reaction, in which free radicals react together to produce more and more reacting species (Figure 8.2). In the case of oxidation this involves the production of peroxides and hydroperoxides. These hydroperoxides may then undergo further decomposition to give a range of low molecular weight aldehydes and ketones. Carbonyl compounds of this type usually have characteristically unpleasant smells, which allows their presence to be detected, literally by following one's nose. They can arise not only from the decomposition of drugs but also from the autoxidation of fats, oils and foodstuffs as well as the perishing of rubber and the hardening of paints.

Stage 2   Chain propagation: free radicals are consumed and generated.

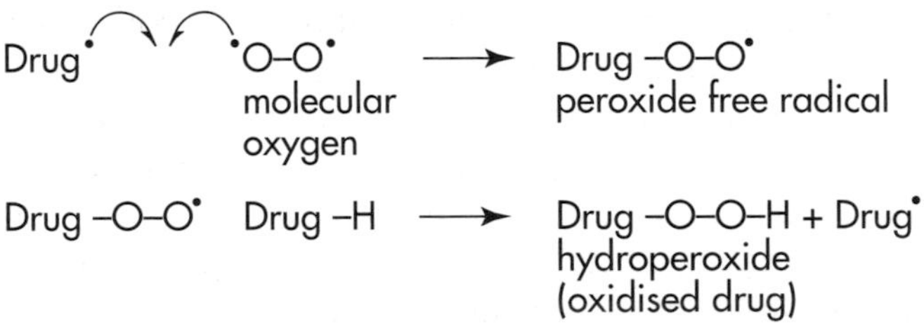

$$\text{Drug}^{\bullet} \quad {}^{\bullet}\text{O--O}^{\bullet} \longrightarrow \text{Drug --O--O}^{\bullet}$$
molecular oxygen   peroxide free radical

$$\text{Drug --O--O}^{\bullet} \quad \text{Drug --H} \longrightarrow \text{Drug --O--O--H} + \text{Drug}^{\bullet}$$
hydroperoxide (oxidised drug)

Figure 8.2   The mechanism of propagation.

Termination

Reactive free radicals join together to form covalent bonds. This effectively ends the chain reaction process and produces stable compounds (Figure 8.3).

Stage 3 **Chain termination:** reactive free radicals are consumed but not generated.

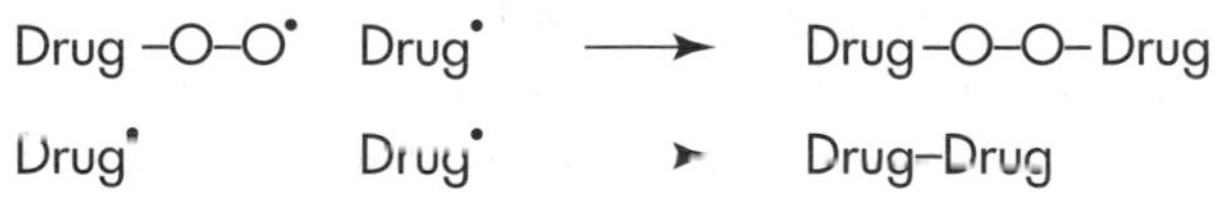

Drug –O–O˙ Drug˙ ⟶ Drug–O–O–Drug

Drug˙   Drug˙   ⟶ Drug–Drug

Figure 8.3 The mechanism of termination.

Stability of free radicals

It is useful to be able to look at the structure of a drug molecule and be able to predict which sites, if any, in the molecule are susceptible to oxidative deterioration. To do this we must have an understanding of the ease of formation and the stability of free radical species.

The most common bond in a drug molecule to be broken during an autoxidation process is a covalent bond between hydrogen and another atom, usually carbon. It follows, therefore, that the more easily this bond undergoes homolysis, the more susceptible the drug will be to autoxidation. See Figure 8.4.

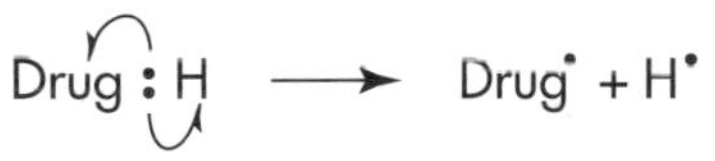

Drug : H ⟶ Drug˙ + H˙

Figure 8.4 Autoxidation of carbon–hydrogen bonds.

The breaking of a bond in this way generates two radicals, each with an unpaired electron. (Note the curved half-arrows in the reaction mechanism. These signify the movement of *one* electron, as opposed to the full arrow found in most reaction schemes, which implies the movement of *two* electrons.) Although almost all free radicals are unstable and react to gain an extra electron to complete a full octet of electrons in their outer electron shell, some radicals are *relatively* more stable than others, and hence will be more likely to form and persist. In general, the more substituted a radical is (with alkyl groups) the more stable it will be, and the more likely it will be to take part in chemical reactions. A rank order can be drawn up that lists the relative stabilities of free radicals; a highly substituted tertiary (3°) radical is considerably more stable than a secondary (2°) or a primary one (1°). The least-stable alkyl radical is the methyl radical, which has no alkyl sub-stituents and therefore no mechanism whereby the unpaired electron can be stabilised:

$$3^y > 2^y > 1^y > CH_3^\bullet$$

Radicals in which the lone electron can be distributed around the molecule by resonance effects are particularly stable and occur in a number of oxidative reaction mechanisms. Examples of comparatively stable radicals of this type are the benzyl free radical and free radicals containing the allyl (or propenyl) group. These species can be stabilised as shown in Figure 8.5.

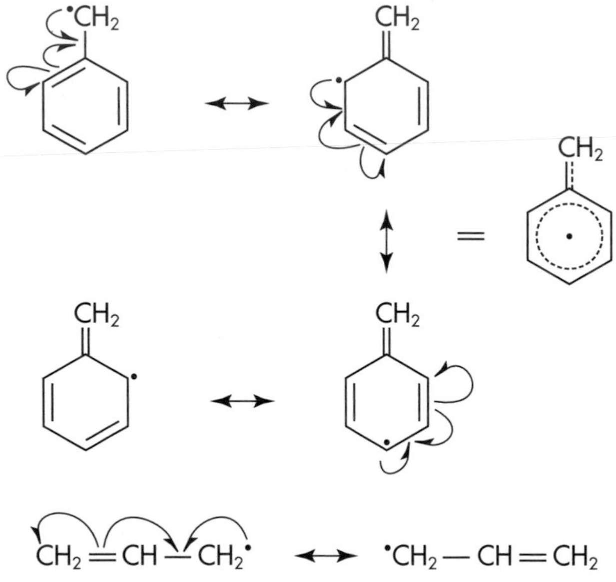

Figure 8.5 The stability of allyl and benzyl radicals.

Drugs that are susceptible to oxidation of carbon–hydrogen bonds include ethers (which oxidise to form highly explosive peroxides), aliphatic amines (which oxidise at the α hydrogen atom) and aldehydes (which are easily oxidised to carboxylic acids and peroxy acids). Examples of these reactions are shown in Figure 8.6.

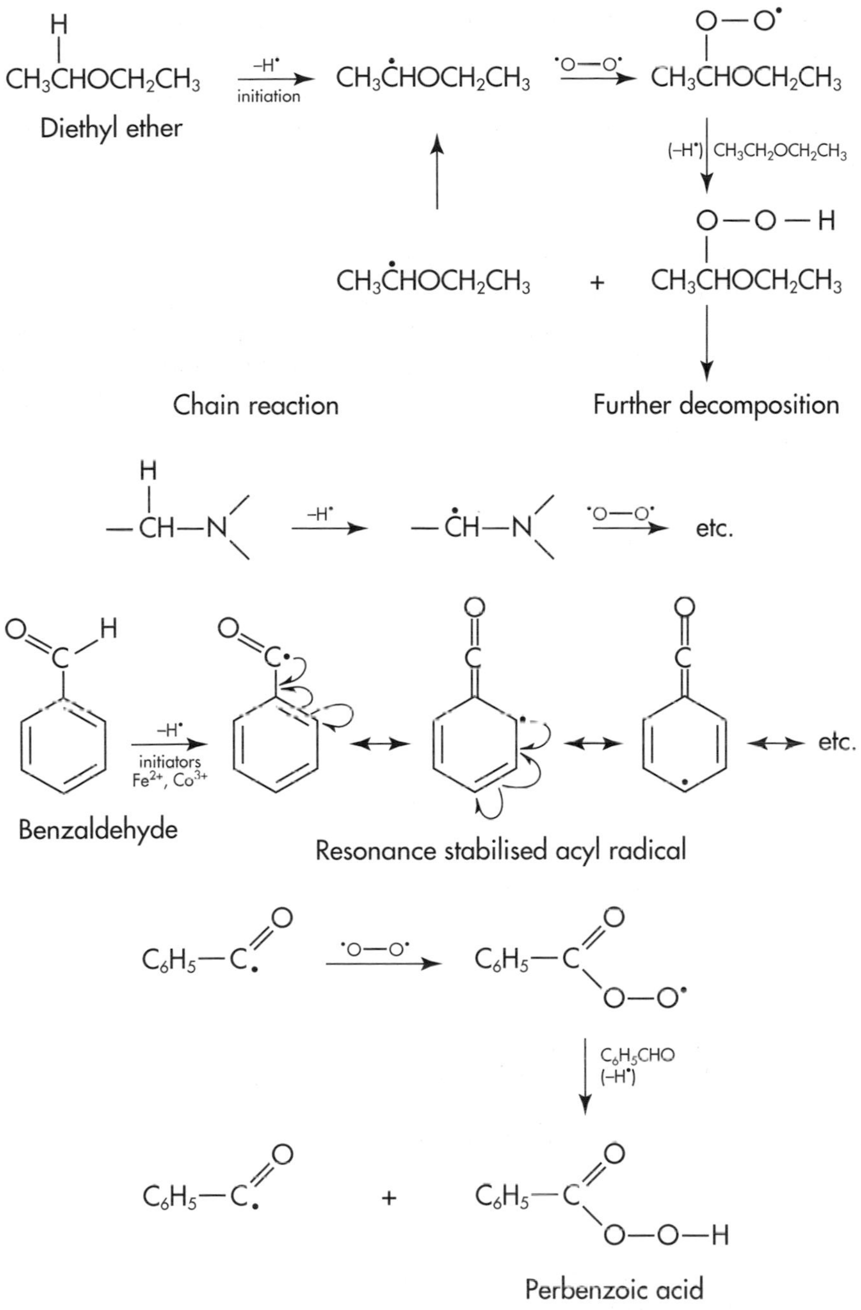

Figure 8.6 Carbon–hydrogen bond cleavage in ethers, amines and aldehydes.

Other bonds that oxidise easily are the oxygen–hydrogen bond found in phenols and the nitrogen–hydrogen bonds found in aromatic amines (Figure 8.7).

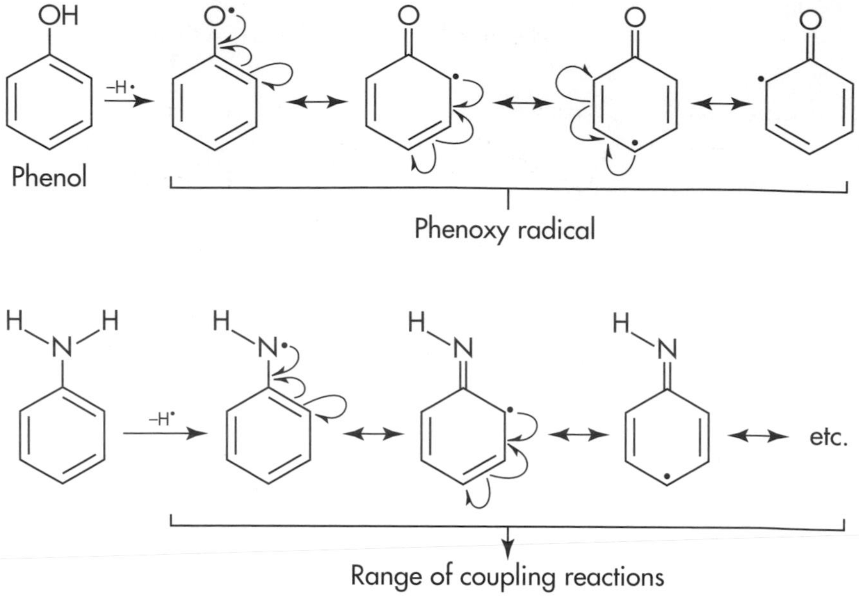

Figure 8.7 Oxygen–hydrogen and nitrogen–hydrogen bond cleavage.

In the case of oxidation of phenols, the reaction can very quickly give a complex mixture of products. This is because the phenoxy radical formed on abstraction of the hydrogen radical, H$^\bullet$ can give rise to carbon–carbon, carbon–oxygen and oxygen–oxygen coupling reactions. The pH at which the phenol is stored is also important since a phenoxide ion, formed at high pH, can easily be oxidised to the phenoxy radical (Figure 8.8).

Drugs containing phenolic groups include the analgesics morphine (and related opiates) and paracetamol as well as the bronchodilator salbutamol, widely used in the treatment of acute asthma. See Figure 8.9.

Drugs that contain two phenolic groups, such as adrenaline (epinephrine) and other catecholamines such as noradrenaline (norepinephrine) and isoprenaline are particularly susceptible to oxidation and have to be formulated at acidic pH. All of these compounds are white crystalline solids, which darken on exposure to air. Adrenaline forms the red coloured compound adrenochrome on oxidation (Figure 8.10),

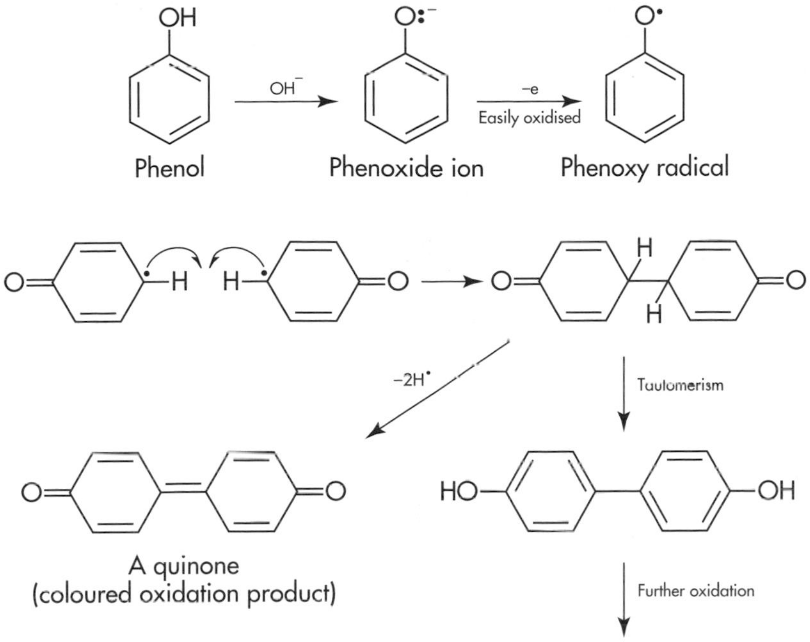

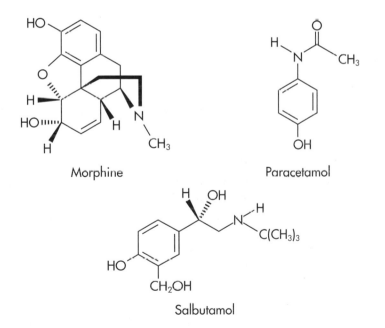

Figure 8.8   Oxidation of the phenoxide ion.

Morphine

Paracetamol

Salbutamol

Figure 8.9   The structures of morphine, paracetamol and salbutamol.

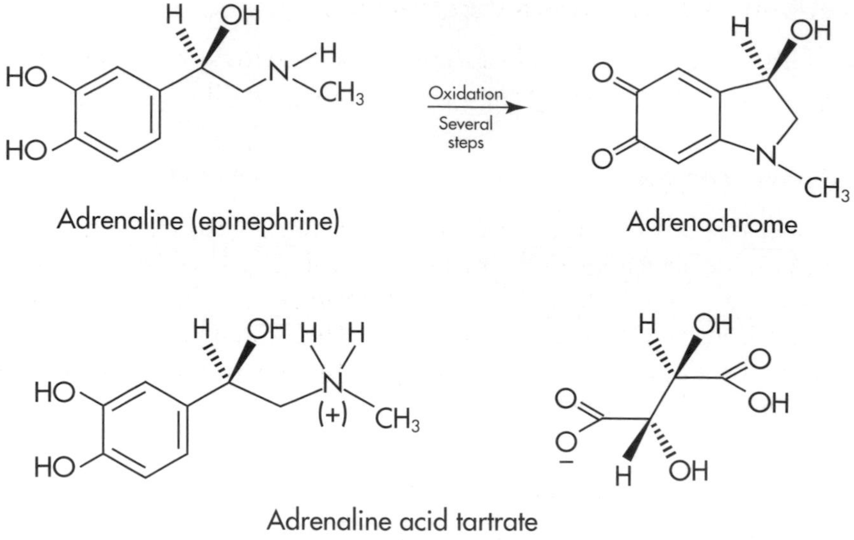

Adrenaline (epinephrine)   Adrenochrome

Adrenaline acid tartrate

Figure 8.10 Oxidation of adrenaline (epinephrine).

which can further polymerise to give black compounds similar in structure to melanin, the natural skin pigment. Injections of adrenaline that develop a pink colour, or that contain crystals of black compound, should not be used for this reason. Adrenaline for injection is formulated as the acid tartrate (Figure 8.10), which, in aqueous solution, gives a pH of approximately 3. It is called the acid tartrate since only one carboxylic acid group of tartaric acid is used up in salt formation with adrenaline. This leaves the remaining carboxylic group to function as an acid.

Cleavage of the nitrogen–hydrogen bond in aromatic amines occurs in a similar manner to that described for phenols, to give a complex mixture of products due to coupling reactions of the type shown in Figure 8.11.

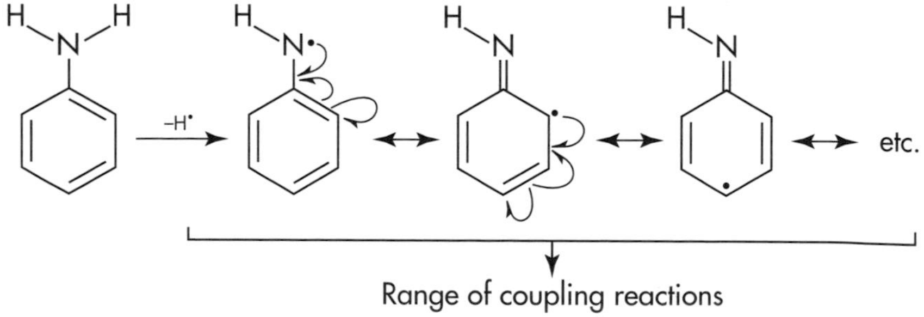

Range of coupling reactions

Figure 8.11 Nitrogen–hydrogen bond cleavage in amines.

Prevention of oxidative deterioration

A number of steps can be taken to minimise oxidative decomposition in drugs and medicines. These can be summarised as follows.

Exclusion of oxygen

This is pretty obvious; if oxygen in the air is causing the oxidation, then exclusion of oxygen from the formulation will minimise oxidative deterioration. This is usually achieved by replacing the oxygen with an inert gas atmosphere (e.g. nitrogen or argon). The container should also be well filled with product and closed tightly to minimise the possibility of air getting to the medicine.

Use of amber or coloured glass containers

Amber glass excludes light of wavelengths <470 nm and so affords some protection to light-sensitive compounds. Special formulations, such as metered dose inhalers used in the treatment of asthma, also offer protection from light and oxygen since the drug is dissolved or suspended in propellant and stored in a sealed aluminium container.

Use of chelating agents

Oxidation reactions can be catalysed by the presence of tiny amounts of metal ions (e.g. 0.05 ppm Cu^{2+} can initiate decomposition of fats) and so stainless steel or glass apparatus should be used wherever possible during manufacture of susceptible compounds. If the presence of metal ions cannot be avoided, then chelating agents, such as disodium edetate, are used to chelate and remove metal ions. Disodium edetate is the disodium salt of ethylenediaminetetraacetic acid, or EDTA, and is shown in Figure 8.12.

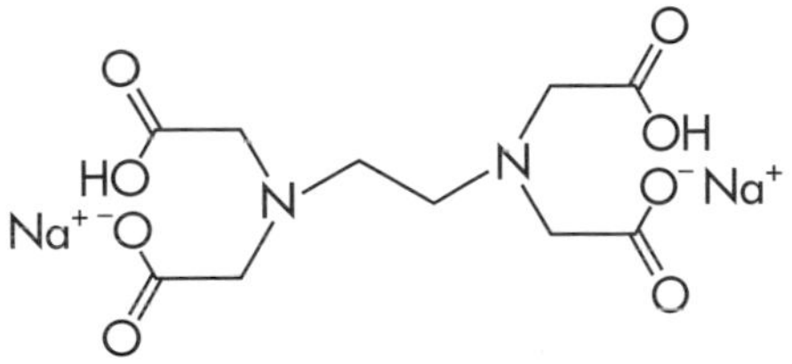

Figure 8.12   The structure of disodium edetate.

Use of antioxidants

Antioxidants are compounds that undergo oxidation easily to form free radicals but which are then not sufficiently reactive to carry on the decomposition chain reaction. They selflessly sacrifice themselves to preserve the drug or medicine. Most antioxidants are phenols and a few of the most commonly used are shown in Figure 8.13.

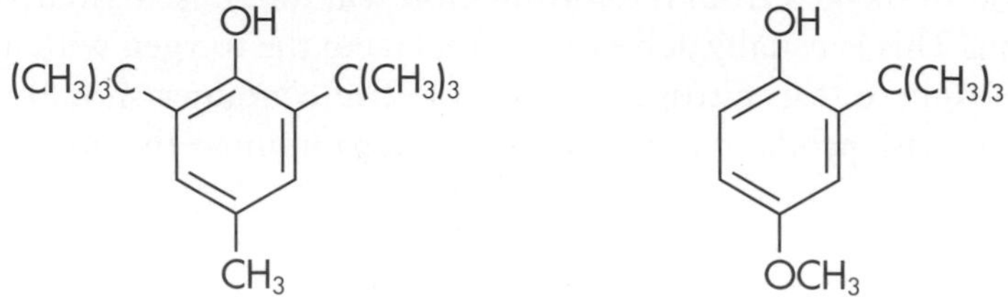

Butylated hydroxytoluene   Butylated hydroxyanisole

Figure 8.13 The structures of butylated hydroxytoluene (BHT) and butylated hydroxyanisole (BHA).

Ascorbic acid (vitamin C) also functions as an antioxidant and is added to medicines and foodstuffs for this reason. Food manufacturers enthusiastically label their products as having 'added vitamin C'. What they are not so keen to tell you is that the vitamin is not there for the consumers' benefit but rather as an antioxidant to stop their product decomposing oxidatively (see Figure 8.14).

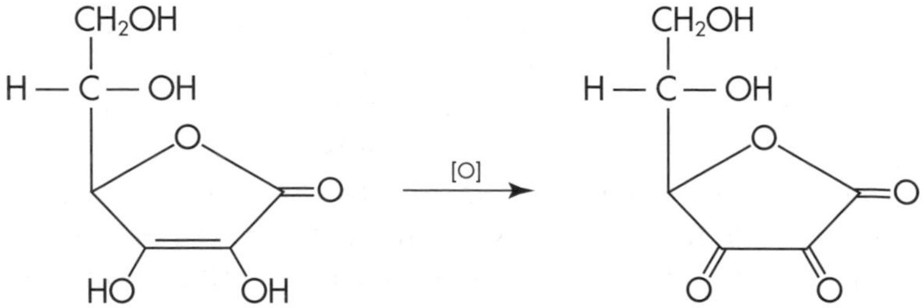

Figure 8.14 The structure of ascorbic acid, showing oxidation to diketone.

Autoxidation of fats and oils

Fixed oils and fats are naturally occuring products, usually of plant origin, that are used extensively in pharmaceutical formulation. They are very susceptible to oxidative decomposition (a process called *rancidity*) and special precautions must be taken to control their stability and prevent their decomposition. Compounds of this type exist as complex mixtures of structurally similar oils, the composition of which can vary from year to year depending on factors such as climate, time of harvest, etc. Chemically, fixed oils and fats are esters of the alcohol glycerol (propane-1,2,3-triol) with three molecules of long-chain carboxylic acids, called fatty acids, which may be the same or different depending on the oil (Figure 8.15).

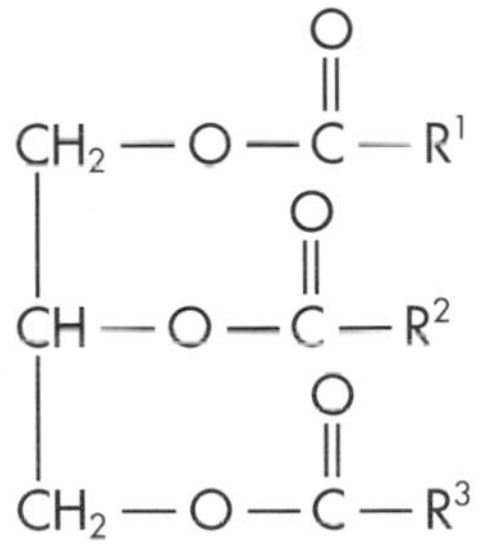

$$
\begin{array}{c}
\quad\quad\quad\quad O \\
\quad\quad\quad\quad \| \\
CH_2 - O - C - R^1 \\
| \quad\quad\quad\quad O \\
| \quad\quad\quad\quad \| \\
CH - O - C - R^2 \\
| \quad\quad\quad\quad O \\
| \quad\quad\quad\quad \| \\
CH_2 - O - C - R^3
\end{array}
$$

Figure 8.15   The structure of triglycerides.

Compounds of this type are called *triglycerides* and contain several sites within the molecule where autoxidation can occur to cause breakdown of the molecule. This is especially true if the fatty acids are *unsaturated* (i.e. contain at least one carbon–carbon double bond; if the carbon chain contains several double bonds, the oil is said to be *polyunsaturated*). The stability of oils is very important in pharmaceuticals since non-polar drugs (for example, contraceptive steroids and neuroleptic tranquillisers) are often formulated in oily injection vehicles for intramuscular or depot injection. Injections of this type can be given, for example, once a month, and the drug exerts its pharmacological effect as it leaches out of the injection site into the bloodstream. Oils used as injection vehicles include arachis oil, from the peanut plant, olive oil, castor oil and ethyl oleate, the ethyl ester of the 18-carbon fatty acid oleic acid (Figure 8.16).

These oils, if they are to be used parenterally, need to be chemically pure and free from microbial contamination. As stated above, plant oils are often complex mixtures of chemically similar compounds and so require special forms of pharmaceutical assay (e.g. determination of their acid and saponification values) as well as physical methods of assay such as determination of density (i.e. weight per millilitre) and measurement of their refractive index. Increasingly, modern instrumental methods of

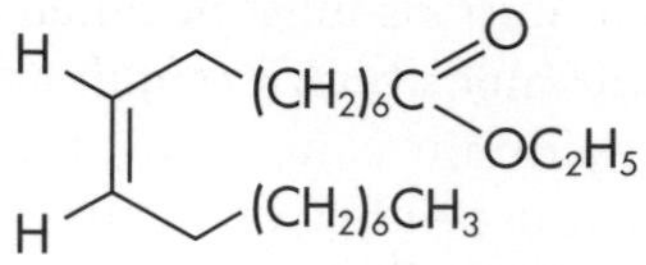

Figure 8.16 The structure of ethyl oleate.

analysis (e.g. gas chromatography) are being used to identify component oils and ensure purity (e.g. see the BP assay of Arachis Oil).

Ageing

The effects of oxygen are not limited only to the oxidation of small molecules found in drugs and medicines. It is now thought that most of the chemical effects of human ageing are as a result of sustained and cumulative oxidative damage on important macromolecules present in our cells (particularly DNA). The old joke to the effect that air is poisonous – everyone who breathes the stuff dies – does have some truth in it. As soon as we are born, the cells in our bodies begin to suffer damage from reactive oxygen species (such as hydroxyl and superoxide radicals). These reactive species are formed by the breakdown of oxygen present in all our cells and, once formed, can react with essential cell components such as phospholipid membranes, cellular proteins and DNA. Damage to DNA results in genetic mutations, which can be passed on to subsequent generations of cells. If the oxidative damage is severe, the cell in question will enter a programme of cell death, called *apoptosis*, and effectively commit suicide.

To counteract these onslaughts by reactive forms of oxygen, the body has evolved a number of elegant defence mechanisms. Repair enzymes can detect damaged DNA bases and repair them *in situ* without disrupting the function of the DNA. Similarly, damaged membrane is repaired to restore cell integrity. These repair enzymes are essentially catalysing an intracellular REDOX process and require a number of essential nutrients such as vitamins C and E to act as antioxidants. The ageing effects of oxidative damage cannot be reversed (yet!) and no amount of expensive cosmetic preparations will stop skin from ageing, but the amount of damage to cells may be reduced by an adequate intake of vitamins and antioxidants in the diet. The most recent nutritional advice is to consume at least three or four helpings of fresh fruit and vegetables every day to maintain an adequate dietary intake of essential antioxidants. It is a sad reflection on our society that much more time, money and advertising are spent on expensive cosmetic 'remedies' for ageing than are spent ensuring a healthy diet for all in the population.

Hydrolysis

Hydrolysis, in its widest sense, is the breaking of a chemical bond due to the reaction of water. This contrasts with *hydration*, which is the addition of the elements of water to a multiple bond, but with no associated fragmentation of the molecule. A large number of functional groups found in drugs are prone to hydrolysis on storage (see Figure 8.17), but the most commonly encountered are esters and amides.

The hydrolysis of esters and amides occurs as a result of nucleophilic attack on the carbon of the carbonyl group and subsequent cleavage of the carbon–oxygen or carbon–nitrogen single bond. The carbon of the carbonyl group is more positive than expected as a result of the high electronegativity of the adjacent oxygen. The unequal sharing of the bond electrons causes a polarisation of the bond so that the carbon bears a partial positive charge (δ^+), while the oxygen has a partial negative charge (δ^-).

Hydrolysis reactions occur quite slowly, but, in the presence of acid or alkali, the rate of the reaction increases and significant decomposition can occur. It should be remembered that many drugs are amines, which can be rendered water-soluble by formation of their hydrochloride salt. Salts of weak bases and strong mineral acids are acidic by partial hydrolysis (see Chapter 1 if this is not familiar) and the H^+ formed by hydrolysis of the salt can catalyse hydrolysis reactions on the drug itself. Similarly, drugs that are salts of weak acids with strong bases are alkaline in solution and the OH^- produced by partial hydrolysis of the salt can act as a catalyst and bring about decomposition. The mechanisms of acid- and base-catalysed hydrolysis of esters are shown in Figures 8.18 and 8.19; the mechanisms for hydrolysis of amides are similar.

Acid-catalysed hydrolysis

The initial protonation on the carbonyl oxygen produces a resonance-stabilised cation; this increases the electrophilicity of the carbonyl group, making it susceptible to attack by the nucleophilic water (Figure 8.18).

Proton transfer from the water to the alcohol converts the latter into a better leaving group (G). Incidentally, this mechanism is the reverse of the mechanism for formation of an ester from an acid and an alcohol under acidic conditions (esterification).

Group	Name	Examples
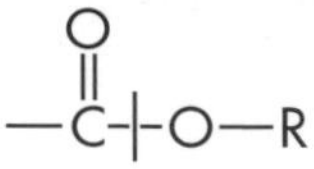	ester	ethyl oleate, aspirin, procaine
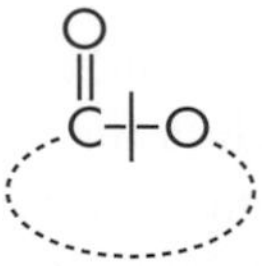	cyclic ester	warfarin, nystatin, digoxin, digitoxin
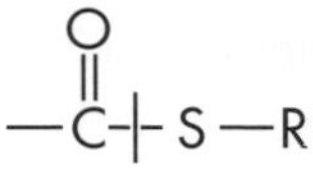	thioester	spironolactone
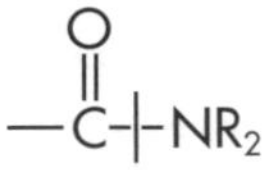	amide	nicotinamide, paracetamol, procainamide
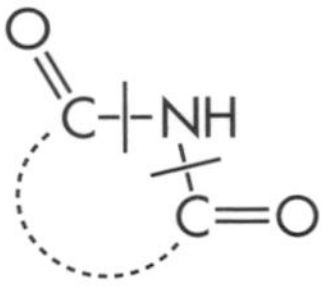	imide	phenytoin, barbiturates, riboflavin
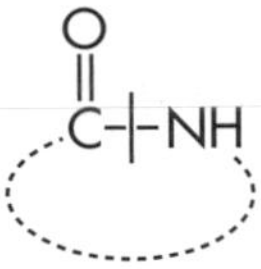	cyclic amide (lactam)	penicillins, cephalosporins
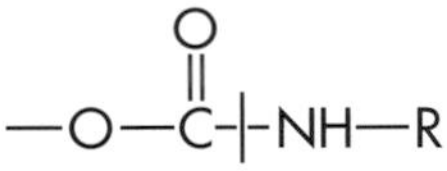	carbamate (urethane)	carbachol, neostigmine, carbimazole
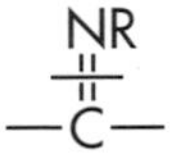	imine (azomethine or Schiffs base)	diazepam, pralidoxime
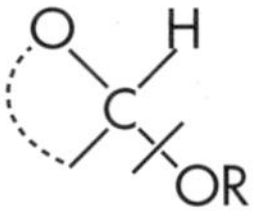	acetal	digoxin, aldosterone
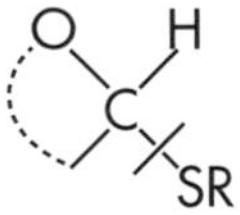	thioacetal	lincomycin, clindamycin
$R-O-SO_3H$	sulfate ester	heparin
$R-NH-SO_3H$	sulfamate	
$R-O-PO_3H$	phosphate ester	hydrocortisone sodium phosphate, triclofos sodium

Figure 8.17 Functional groups prone to hydrolysis.

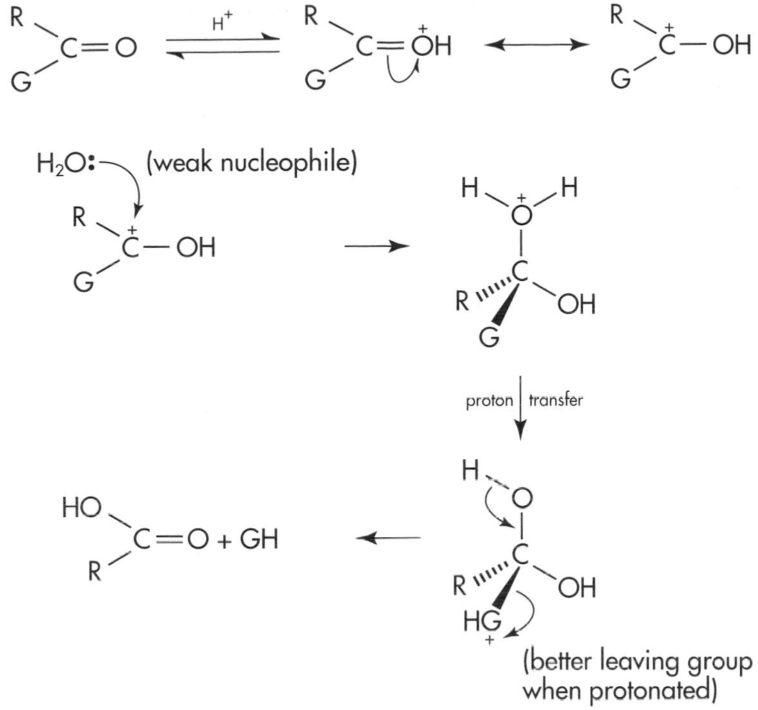

Figure 8.18   The mechanism of acid-catalysed hydrolysis.

Base-catalysed hydrolysis

This reaction is easier to follow; the nucleophile in this case is the strongly basic OH⁻ ion, which attacks the δ^+ carbon of the carbonyl group directly (Figure 8.19).

Note that in base-catalysed hydrolysis the acid formed by hydrolysis instantaneously reacts with the excess of base to form the salt of the

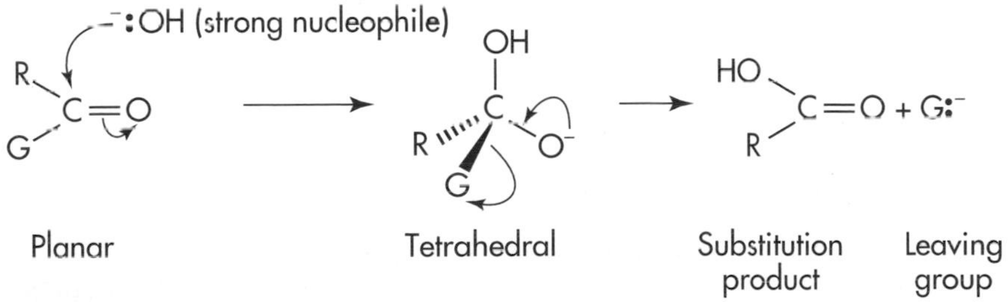

Figure 8.19   The mechanism of base-catalysed hydrolysis.

acid. The free acid may be obtained, if desired, by acidification of the mixture.

Examples of drugs susceptible to hydrolysis

Figure 8.17 lists examples of the types of drugs containing functional groups prone to decomposition by hydrolysis. There is insufficient space to consider each drug in detail, but a few important examples will be considered.

Aspirin

Aspirin, the widely used analgesic, is the acetyl ester of salicylic acid and is very susceptible to hydrolysis; moisture in the air is sufficient to bring about significant decomposition. A bottle of aspirin tablets almost always smells of vinegar when opened; this is due to the reaction shown in Figure 8.20 taking place to liberate salicylic and acetic acids. The decomposition is increased when members of the public store aspirin tablets in the bathroom cabinet, the one room in the house that is guaranteed to have a hot, steamy atmosphere ideal for hydrolysis reactions.

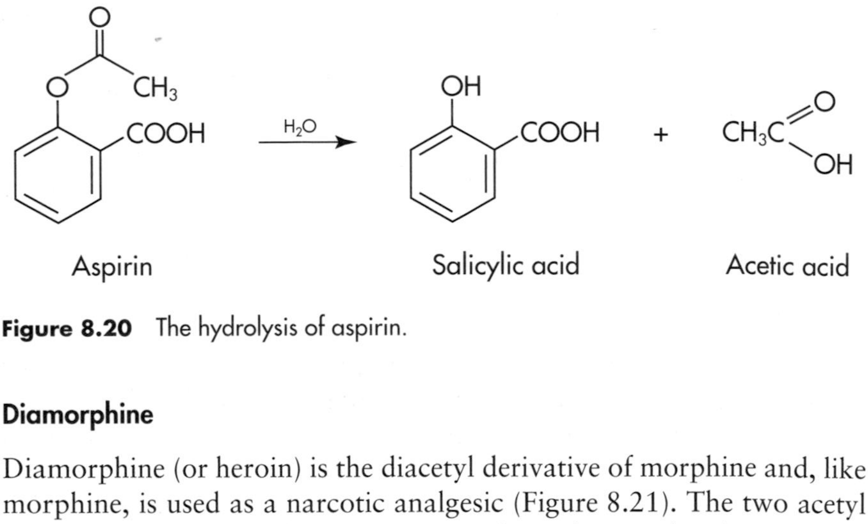

| Aspirin | Salicylic acid | Acetic acid |

Figure 8.20 The hydrolysis of aspirin.

Diamorphine

Diamorphine (or heroin) is the diacetyl derivative of morphine and, like morphine, is used as a narcotic analgesic (Figure 8.21). The two acetyl groups are important for two reasons; first, they render the molecule more lipophilic (increasing the partition coefficient), which means that diamorphine is absorbed into the central nervous system more rapidly than is morphine, and in turn results in a faster onset of action than for morphine (and, sadly, makes the compound a favourite with addicts).

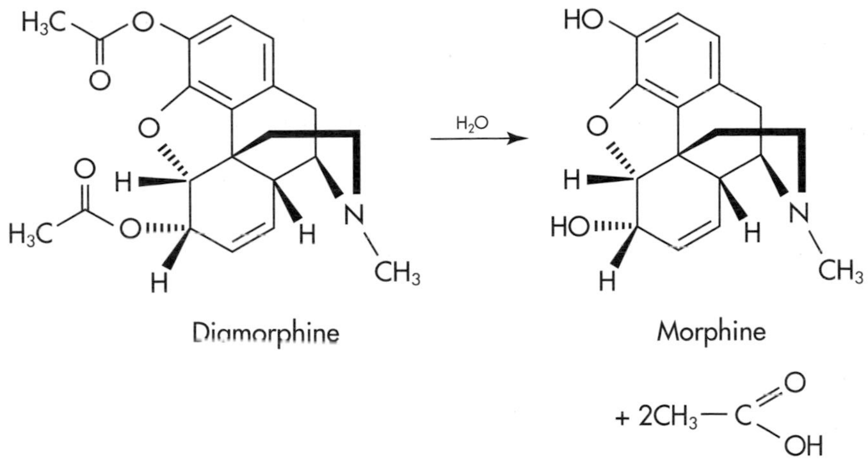

Figure 8.21 The structure and hydrolysis of diamorphine.

The second aspect of the two acetyl groups is that they are susceptible to hydrolysis, to yield morphine and two molecules of acetic acid (Figure 8.21).

Diamorphine injection is prepared by dissolving the contents of a sealed container in Water for Injections BP immediately prior to use. The instability of the ester groups precludes sterilisation of the injection by autoclaving.

A close inspection of the structure of diamorphine will show that the molecule also contains 'benzylic' hydrogen atoms, on the CH_2 adjacent to the benzene ring. This site is susceptible to oxidation and, for this reason, diamorphine should be stored in a well-closed container protected from light.

Penicillin

Penicillin (and, for that matter cephalosporin) antibiotics are cyclic amides and are very prone to hydrolysis. Normal amide bonds are more resistant to hydrolysis than are esters, but in penicillins the amide is cyclised into a four-membered β-lactam ring. The bond angles in this ring are close to 90°, in contrast to an open-chain amide in which the bond angle is 120° (sp^2 hybridised carbon). This unnatural bond angle in the β-lactam ring means that the ring is very easily opened by nucleophiles, particularly water.

The effect is compounded by the geometry of the fused bicyclic ring system. The β-lactam and thiazolidine rings of penicillin do not lie in the same plane (in fact, they lie almost perpendicular to each other), so resonance effects within the cyclic amide are prevented, which leaves the carbonyl carbon atom much more δ^+ than expected and hence more liable to nucleophilic attack. The structures of a penicillin (ampicillin) and the decomposition product, penicilloic acid, are shown in Figure 8.22.

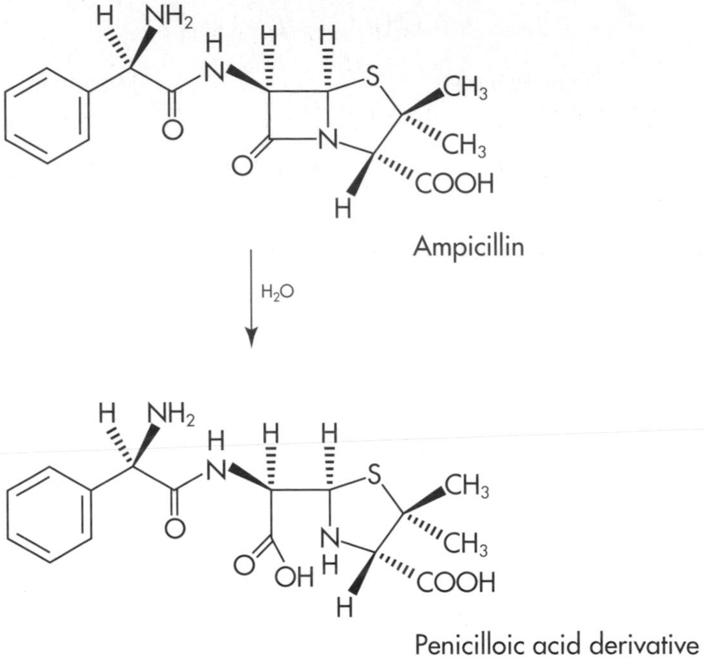

Ampicillin

H_2O

Penicilloic acid derivative

Figure 8.22   The structures of ampicillin and penicilloic acid.

Penicillin and cephalosporin antibiotics are insufficiently stable to be supplied dissolved in aqueous solutions. Instead, they are supplied as a dry powder, which is reconstituted immediately prior to dispensing by the pharmacist. The solution (or, more accurately, suspension) dispensed must be stored in a refrigerator and discarded after 7 days. The ring-opened product (penicilloic acid) is inactive as an antibiotic.

Other mechanisms of degradation

Rarely, some other forms of decomposition may be encountered. These include hydration (found in some alkaloids of ergot), polymerisation (which can affect solutions of the antibiotic ampicillin) and dimerisation reactions (which can be seen as a result of free radical attack on morphine). While these methods of decomposition are important and should be borne in mind, the majority of chemical deterioration can be explained by consideration of the few mechanisms outlined above.

Tutorial examples

Q   *1   Predict which of the following fatty acids will undergo oxidation most easily, and explain what precautions should be employed to minimise the oxidation.*

$CH_3(CH_2)_6CH_2CH=CHCH_2(CH_2)_6COOH$ *(oleic acid)*

$CH_3(CH_2)_3CH_2CH=CHCH_2CH=CHCH_2(CH_2)_6COOH$
(linoleic acid)

$CH_3CH_2CH=CHCH_2CH=CHCH_2CH=CHCH_2(CH_2)_6COOH$
(linolenic acid)

A   1   Compounds that contain allylic and benzylic centres are especially prone to autoxidation, since the radicals formed on oxidation are stabilised by resonance. Oleic acid contains two allylic positions, linoleic acid contains two allylic positions and one 'double allylic' position, while linolenic contains two allylic and two 'double allylic' positions. We would therefore expect linolenic to be the most susceptible acid to oxidation, followed by linoleic and oleic. (The actual relative rates of autoxidation are linolenic (25) > linoleic (12) > oleic (1)).

Precautions that can be employed to minimise oxidative deterioration are reducing the oxygen concentration in the container by, for example, the use of an inert atmosphere, and the use of a well-closed and well-filled container. It would also be advisable to store the product at low temperature and in a dark place.

Q   *2   The BP monograph for Chloramphenicol Eye Drops contains a limit test for 2-amino-1-(4-nitrophenyl)propane-1,3-diol (Figure 8.23).*
(a)   Explain why this limit test is included, and show how the diol could be formed.
(b)   Both chloramphenicol and the diol absorb ultraviolet light at the same λ_{max}. Outline the principles of a stability-indicating test that could be used to measure the amount of diol in the eye drops.

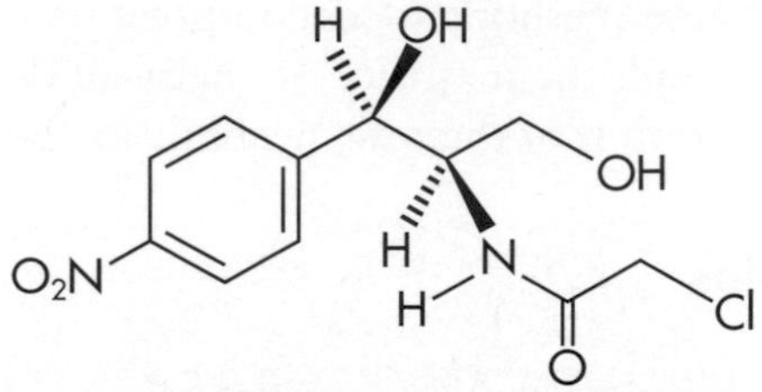

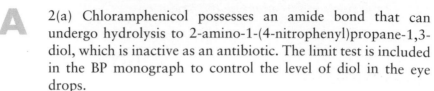

Figure 8.23 The structure of chloramphenicol.

2(a) Chloramphenicol possesses an amide bond that can undergo hydrolysis to 2-amino-1-(4-nitrophenyl)propane-1,3-diol, which is inactive as an antibiotic. The limit test is included in the BP monograph to control the level of diol in the eye drops.

(b) Since both compounds have the same chromophore, they will absorb ultraviolet radiation of the same wavelength. They must therefore be separated from each other and measured individually, otherwise an ultraviolet assay will be unable to determine the extent of deterioration. This separation may easily be accomplished by addition of dilute hydrochloric acid solution to the eye drops. The diol is basic and will ionise to form the hydrochloride salt. Extraction with an organic solvent removes the neutral chloramphenicol, leaving the salt in the aqueous phase, which can easily be measured spectrophotometrically. A chromatographic technique, such as high performance liquid chromatography (HPLC), would also allow determination of the diol in the presence of chloramphenicol. Here the separation is achieved on an HPLC column and each compound enters the UV detector individually.

Problems

Q8.1 Novobiocin is an antibiotic, formerly used in the treatment of infections caused by Gram-positive organisms (Figure 8.24).

(a) Identify and name the functional groups that are likely to undergo oxidation on storage.

(b) Identify and name the functional groups that are susceptible to hydrolysis.

(c) What conditions would you recommend for the storage of novobiocin?

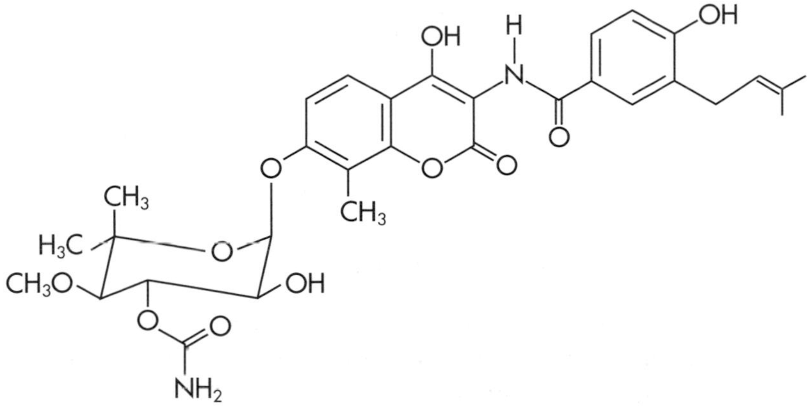

Figure 8.24 The structure of novobiocin.

(d) When novobiocin was mixed with 5% Dextrose Injection, the solution became cloudy. Account for this observation.

Q8.2 Explain each of the following observations. Your answer should include appropriate chemical formulae.

(a) Penicillin suspensions are supplied as dried granules and are reconstituted by the pharmacist immediately prior to use.
(b) Solutions of adrenaline (epinephrine) become pink on exposure to sunlight.
(c) Samples of aspirin tablets invariably smell of vinegar.
(d) The vasoconstrictor peptide angiotensin II has a very short half-life within the body.

(Answers to problems can be found on pp. 224–227.)

9

Kinetics of drug stability

The routes of decomposition of drugs, and the steps taken to prevent them, were considered in Chapter 8. In this chapter the rates of decomposition will be studied and useful information, such as shelf-life, will be predicted. Calculations of this type are important as there is little merit in producing the latest wonderdrug designed to cure all ills only to watch it fall apart on the dispensary shelf as a result of decomposition.

Rate, order and molecularity

The underlying principle on which all of the science of kinetics is built is the law of mass action introduced in Chapter 1. This states that the rate of a chemical reaction (i.e. the speed of the reaction or, simply, how fast it is) is proportional to the active masses of the reacting substances. Active mass is a complicated term to measure, but, fortunately, if the solutions in question are dilute, the active mass may be replaced by concentration, which is much easier to handle. If the concentration of a solute is greater than about 0.1 mol L^{-1}, significant interactions arise between the solute molecules or ions. In cases like this, effective and measured concentrations are not the same and use must be made of *activity* instead of concentration.

The rate of a chemical reaction is, in a dilute solution, proportional to the concentrations of the various reactants each raised to the power of the number of moles of the reactant in the balanced chemical equation. This sounds too easy, and in fact it is. In practice, the rate of a chemical reaction depends only on a small number of concentration terms, and the sum of the powers to which these concentrations are raised is termed the *order* of the reaction. This is because chemical reactions occur in a number of steps, or stages (called a *mechanism*) and the rate of the overall reaction is often governed by the rate of the slowest step (called, not surprisingly, the *rate-determining step*). Even if every other stage of a chemical reaction occurs instantaneously, the rate of the reaction as a whole cannot exceed that of the slowest stage.

For example, if the rate of a chemical reaction depended only on the concentration of compound A, this could be written as

Rate $\propto$ [A]

and the reaction would be *first order*, e.g.

$$C_2H_6 \rightleftharpoons C_2H_4 + H_2$$

If the rate of the reaction depended on the concentrations of A and B, or on the concentration of A squared, this could be written as

Rate $\propto$ [A][B]   or   Rate $\propto$ [A]^2

and the reaction would be *second order*, e.g.

$$CH_3COOC_2H_5 + NaOH \rightleftharpoons C_2H_5OH + CH_3COONa$$

To further complicate matters, the order of a chemical reaction cannot be predicted from the chemical equation, even if it has been balanced. The order of a reaction is determined *experimentally* from accurate measurements of the rate under different conditions. It is possible for reactions to be third order, zero order (often found in solid-state reactions such as the release of drug from pharmaceutical suspensions) or even of a fractional order.

The third term to be considered in this section is *molecularity*. The molecularity of a reaction is the total number of molecules taking part in the slowest of the elementary reaction steps. In most chemical reactions, two molecules collide and react; the molecularity is 2 and the reaction is said to be *bimolecular*. Reactions in which only one molecule is involved (*unimolecular*) are known, but usually occur only in the gas phase. Reactions with a molecularity higher than 2 are very rare, since this would require three or more reactants all encountering each other at the same time.

Rate equations and first-order reactions

Differential rate equations like the ones above are not much use to the practising chemist, so it is usual to integrate the rate equation to obtain more useful expressions. This can be carried out as follows for a first-order reaction. In this reaction, compound A reacts to form products. At the start of the reaction (time 0) the concentration of A is equal to a mol L^{-1}, while the concentration of products will be zero (since the reaction has not started). At some later time, t, the concentration of products has increased to x mol L^{-1} and as a result the concentration of A has fallen to $(a - x)$ mol L^{-1}. This can be represented mathematically as

$A \longrightarrow$ products

At time = 0,

$[A] = a$, $\qquad [\text{products}] = 0$

At time = t,

$[A] = (a - x)$, $\qquad [\text{products}] = x$

From the law of mass action, the rate of reaction is proportional to $[A]$.

If we rewrite 'rate' as dx/dt, i.e. the rate of production of x with respect to t, and substituting $(a - x)$ for $[A]$, then

$$\frac{dx}{dt} \propto (a - x)$$

and so

$$\frac{dx}{dt} = k(a - x)$$

where k is the constant of proportionality. This expression can be integrated to give

$$\int \frac{dx}{(a - x)} = \int k \, dt = k \int dt$$
$$- \ln(a - x) + c = kt$$

where ln represents the natural (base e) logarithm. To find c, recall that at $t = 0$, $x = 0$; therefore,

$$- \ln a + c = 0$$

and so

$$c = \ln a$$

so that

$$- \ln(a - x) + \ln a = kt$$

or

$$\ln \frac{a}{(a - x)} = kt \tag{9.1}$$

which is equivalent to

$$\ln(a - x) = \ln a - kt \tag{9.2}$$

If a plot of equation (9.1) is made, with t on the horizontal axis and $\ln[a/(a-x)]$ on the vertical axis, a straight line passing through the origin will be obtained for a reaction obeying first-order kinetics. The slope of this straight line will be equal to k the *rate constant* for the reaction (see Figure 9.1).

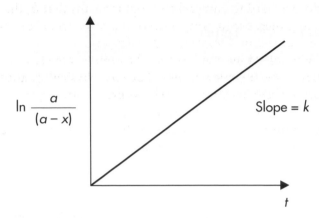

Figure 9.1 Graph of $\ln[a/(a-x)]$ vs t.

For equation (9.2), a plot of $\ln(a-x)$ vs t will yield a straight line the slope of which is negative and equal to $-k$, and the intercept with the vertical axis equal to $\ln a$ (see Figure 9.2).

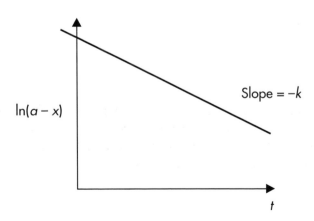

Figure 9.2 Graph of $\ln(a-x)$ vs t.

The rate constant, k, is a very important measure of a reaction rate and has the dimension of time^{-1} for a first-order process. This can be shown from equation (9.1), where cancelling terms on the left-hand side of the equation results in no units. The right-hand side of the equation must also have no units if the equation is valid. The term t has the dimension of 'time', so k must have the dimension of time^{-1}. Units of 'inverse time' are hard to comprehend, but it means that k, the rate constant, gives us a measure of how much of the reaction occurs *per unit of time*, i.e. *per second*, or *per hour*, or *per day*, etc.

On a practical point, the fact that the units of concentration cancel out for a first-order reaction means that *any* physical quantity that is *proportional* to the concentration may be used in the equation in place of concentration, e.g. light absorbance or titration volume. This is very useful, since it means data measured in the laboratory can be inserted directly into the integrated rate equation.

Half-life

The half-life $(t_{1/2})$ of a reaction is an important term that may be derived from equation (9.1). The half-life is defined as the time taken for the concentration of reactant to fall to half its original value:

$$\ln \frac{a}{(a-x)} = kt$$

$$\ln \frac{a}{(a - \frac{1}{2}a)} = kt_{1/2}$$

$$\ln 2 = kt_{1/2}$$

$$t_{1/2} = \frac{0.693}{k} \tag{9.3}$$

For first-order reactions (only), $t_{1/2}$ is independent of concentration. This means that the time taken for the reactant concentration to fall from 1 M to 0.5 M will be the same as the time taken to fall from 0.5 M to 0.25 M. This is *not* true for higher orders of reaction.

Shelf-life

The shelf life (t_{90}) of a pharmaceutical product is the length of time the product may safely be stored on the dispensary shelf before significant decomposition occurs. This is important since, at best, drugs may decompose to inactive products; in the worst case the decomposition may yield toxic compounds. The shelf-life is often taken to be the time for decomposition of 10% of the active drug to occur, leaving 90% of the activity. A similar expression to equation (9.3) can be obtained by substituting $\ln(100/90)$ in place of $\ln 2$ to give

$$t_{90} = \frac{0.105}{k} \tag{9.4}$$

from which the shelf-life can easily be calculated once k, the reaction rate constant, has been determined.

Second-order reactions

For reactions of the type

$$2A \longrightarrow \text{products} \qquad \text{or} \qquad A + B \longrightarrow \text{products}$$

the rate of the reaction will be first order with respect to each reactant and hence second order overall. A useful integrated rate equation may be obtained by a similar process to the derivation of equation (9.1) as follows:

$$\frac{dx}{dt} = k(a - x)^2$$

Therefore,

$$\int \frac{dx}{(a - x)^2} = \int k \, dt$$

Hence,

$$\frac{1}{(a - x)} + c = kt$$

At $t = 0$, $x = 0$, therefore $1/a + c = 0$ and $c = -1/a$ to give

$$\frac{1}{(a - x)} - \frac{1}{a} = kt \tag{9.5}$$

Equation (9.5) is the equation of a straight line of the type $y - c = mx$, so that a plot of $1/(a - x)$ against t yields a straight line of slope k, with an intercept on the vertical axis of $1/a$.

Equation (9.5) is valid for second-order reactions in which the concentrations of the reactants are equal. A general second-order equation may also be derived that will apply to reactions of the type $A + B \rightarrow$ products when [A] does not equal [B], but this is outside the scope of this book. In most cases it is possible to arrange for the concentrations of the reactants to be equal and equation (9.5) may be used.

The term k is, again, the rate constant for the reaction, but in a second-order process k has dimensions of concentration^{-1} time^{-1}. The relationship between the half-life and the second-order rate constant, k, for initial equal concentrations of reactant can be found by substituting $t = t_{1/2}$ into equation (9.5) as follows:

$$\frac{1}{(a-x)} - \frac{1}{a} = kt$$

$$\frac{1}{(a-\frac{1}{2}a)} - \frac{1}{a} = kt_{1/2}$$

$$\frac{1}{\frac{1}{2}a} - \frac{1}{a} = kt_{1/2}$$

$$\frac{1}{a} = kt_{1/2}$$

$$t_{1/2} = \frac{1}{ak} \tag{9.6}$$

Since k is a constant, the half-life of a second-order reaction where the initial reactant concentrations are equal is inversely proportional to a, the initial reactant concentration.

In some second-order reactions the concentration of one of the reactants is many times more than the concentration of the other, so large in fact as to be considered constant throughout the reaction. In these cases, the reaction appears to follow first-order kinetics, even though, strictly speaking, it is still a second-order process. Reactions such as these are termed *pseudo first-order* reactions. A good example is the acid- or base-catalysed hydrolysis of an ester, in which the concentration of water is so large compared to the concentration of ester as to be considered constant. The rate of the hydrolysis appears to vary only with the concentration of the ester.

Zero-order reactions

There are some reactions in which the rate of the reaction is independent of the concentration of the reactants but does depend on some other factor, such as the amount of catalyst present. These reactions are termed *zero-order* reactions, and rate equations can be derived as follows:

$$\frac{\mathrm{d}x}{\mathrm{d}t} = k[\mathrm{A}]^0$$

Therefore,

$$\int \mathrm{d}x = \int k\,\mathrm{d}t$$

which gives

$$x = kt + c \tag{9.7}$$

In zero-order reactions the amount of product formed varies with time so that the amount of product formed after 20 minutes will be twice that formed after 10 minutes. Reactions that follow zero-order kinetics are quite rare, but they do occur in solid-phase reactions such as release of drug from a pharmaceutical suspension.

Reaction rates and temperature

For most chemical reactions an increase in temperature will bring about an associated increase in reaction rate, which can be measured by an increase in k, the reaction rate constant. As a very rough guide, an increase in temperature of 10 °C will approximately double the rate of a reaction.

The Swedish chemist Arrhenius first expressed mathematically the relationship between reaction rate and temperature, namely,

$$k = A\mathrm{e}^{-E/RT} \tag{9.8}$$

where A is a constant known as the *frequency factor* and is a measure of the number of collisions taking place between reactants; $\mathrm{e}^{-E/RT}$ is the small fraction of the total number of collisions that result in a successful reaction; E is the activation energy for the reaction, i.e. the energy required to force the reactants to collide with enough energy to form a product; R is the universal gas constant ($R = 8.314\ \mathrm{J\ K^{-1}\ mol^{-1}}$), which seems to crop up in almost every physical chemistry equation; and T is the temperature in kelvin.

Taking logarithms of equation (9.8) gives

$$\ln k = \ln A - \frac{E}{RT} \tag{9.9}$$

which is instantly recognisable as the equation of a straight line
($y = c - mx$). This means that if the reaction rate, k, is determined at a
number of temperatures, a graph of $\ln k$ against $1/T$ (T in kelvin) will
yield a straight line of slope $-E/R$ and intersect the vertical axis at $\ln A$.
The activation energy, E, for the reaction may be determined from data
like these.

Even more usefully, if the reaction rate k_1 is determined at a
temperature T_1, and the rate k_2 is determined at a temperature T_2, then
the two forms of equation (9.9) may be subtracted to give

$$\ln \frac{k_2}{k_1} = -\frac{E}{R}\left(\frac{1}{T_2} - \frac{1}{T_1}\right) \tag{9.10}$$

This useful equation may be used to predict the reaction rate at any temperature once k_1 and E are known for temperature T_1. This type of calculation is extremely important in pharmaceutical science since it is used
to predict shelf-life for medicines. Once a medicine has been manufac-
tured, it is stored under high-stress conditions (e.g. at elevated temperature, high humidity, under strong lighting, etc.) and the rates of
decomposition are measured and the activation energy is calculated.
From these data, the value of k may be predicted and the likely shelf-life
for the medicine can be calculated for room temperature (25 °C) or
refrigerator temperature (4 °C). Another useful point to notice is that
since k enters into the graphs as $\ln k$, and into the equations as a ratio,
any physical quantity that is proportional to k, such as the actual
reaction rates at fixed concentrations of reactants, may be used in the
equation instead of k.

Calculations using *Arrhenius plots*, such as those described above,
are carried out in the pharmaceutical industry every day. It should be
made clear, however, that they involve a number of assumptions. It is
assumed that the linearity of the graph obtained from equation (9.9)
extends to room temperature, or, mathematically, that A and E are independent of temperature. If the line cannot be extrapolated to room temperature, shelf-life predictions are invalid. Second, it is assumed that the
same chemical reaction is occurring with decomposition at high temperature as at low temperature. This is usually the case, but until proven it
remains an assumption in most calculations.

Tutorial example

Q   1   *The reaction between aspirin and gastric acid may be followed by titrating the liberated salicylic and acetic acids with sodium hydroxide. In an experiment using equimolar amounts of reactants, the following data were obtained:*

Time (s)	0	89	208	375	625	803
[Aspirin] (mol L^{-1})	1.6	1.4	1.2	1.0	0.8	0.7

Determine the order of the reaction and determine the rate constant.

A   1   The order of a chemical reaction cannot be determined by inspection, it must be determined experimentally. In practice, this means measuring the decomposition of the compound under controlled conditions and applying each of the rate equations in turn to see which type of equation fits the data and gives the best straight line. This is what scientists term an empirical method, and what the man in the street calls 'trial and error'!

In the case of the hydrolysis of aspirin, it would be sensible to try the second-order rate equation first (especially since the question stresses that the reactant concentrations are equal).

For a second-order process, equation (9.5) is valid, i.e.

$$\frac{1}{(a-x)} - \frac{1}{a} = kt$$

where $(a - x)$ is the concentration of each reactant at time t, and a plot of $1/(a - x)$ vs t should yield a straight line of slope k.

This plot was carried out and a straight line was obtained with a slope of 1.0×10^{-3}. This proves that the reaction is second order with a rate constant, $k = 1.0 \times 10^{-3}$ (mol L^{-1})$^{-1}$ s^{-1}.

Problems

Q9.1   Determine the first-order rate constant for the hydrolysis of acetyl-β-methylcholine at 85 °C from the information given below.

[Drug] (mg mL^{-1})	9.35	7.45	4.52	3.46	1.26	0.90
t (days)		0.08	0.75	1.96	2.96	5.75	6.75

Q9.2 (a) Hydrogen peroxide solutions are normally stable, but when metal ions are added, hydrogen peroxide decomposes:

$$2H_2O_2 \rightarrow 2H_2O + O_2$$

In a solution containing $FeCl_3$, the concentration of H_2O_2 varied as follows:

Time (s)	0	27	52	86	121	160	218
[H$_2$O$_2$] (M)	0.80	0.72	0.64	0.56	0.48	0.40	0.32

Using these data, determine the order of the reaction with respect to peroxide, and the value of the rate constant (include appropriate units).

(b) Discuss how you would use kinetic data obtained from monitoring the degradation of a drug to construct an Arrhenius plot. How could you use this plot to determine the frequency factor and activation energy for the reaction?

(c) For a first-order reaction, deduce the units for the frequency factor and activation energy.

(Answers to problems can be found on p. 227.)

10

Answers to problems

A1.1 (a) Ethanolamine is a base since it has an available lone pair of electrons. The compound is a primary aliphatic amine, and a primary alcohol. The pK_a value of 9.4 refers to the ionisation of the conjugate acid of ethanolamine ($HOCH_2CH_2NH_3^+$). Since ethanolamine is a relatively strong organic base, the conjugate acid is a weak acid, therefore has a high pK_a of 9.4.

(b) Since ethanolamine is a base, aqueous solutions of the compound will be alkaline:

$$HOCH_2CH_2NH_2 + H_2O \rightleftharpoons HOCH_2CH_2NH_3^+ + OH^-$$

The base abstracts a proton from water to generate OH^- therefore the solution will be alkaline.

(c) A 1% w/v solution contains 1 g in 100 mL = 10 g in 1000 mL = 10/61.08 mol in 1000 mL = 0.164 mol L^{-1}. Using equation (1.3),

$$pH = pK_w - \tfrac{1}{2}pK_b + \tfrac{1}{2}\log c$$

where $pK_w = 14$, and

$$pK_b = (14 - 9.4) = 4.6$$
$$pH = 11.3$$

which, as predicted, is alkaline.

(d) A solution of ethanolamine (base, B) and its salt (BH^+) will function as a buffer solution. Since the required pH of 9.0 is close to the pK_a value of 9.4, the buffer should be effective over the required range.

$$HOCH_2CH_2NH_2 + HOCH_2CH_2NH_3^+ Cl^-$$

On addition of acid (H^+),

$$B + H^+ \rightleftharpoons BH^+$$

The added strong acid, reacts with the high concentration of free base to give the weaker acid BH^+, therefore little change occurs in pH.

On addition of base (OH^-),

$$BH^+ + OH^- \rightleftharpoons B + H_2O$$

The added strong base reacts with the high concentration of salt to form the weaker base B, therefore little change occurs in pH.

A1.2   (a) pK_a is the negative logarithm to the base 10 of K_a, the acid dissociation constant for the ionisation of the molecule. pK_a can be used to indicate the strength of bases (or, more exactly, the strength of the conjugate acid of the base) since $pK_a + pK_b = 14$.

(b)   The salt formed at the end point of this titration (ephedrine hydrochloride) will be acidic by partial hydrolysis (salt of a weak base and a strong acid); therefore, the pH at the end point can be given by equation (1.2).

$$pH = \tfrac{1}{2}pK_a - \tfrac{1}{2}\log c$$

where c is the concentration of the salt.

$$pH = \tfrac{1}{2}(9.6) - \tfrac{1}{2}\log 0.05$$

(since the volume has doubled, the concentration has halved).

$$pH = 5.45$$

(c)   A possible composition for the buffer would be a mixture of acetic acid and a salt of acetic acid (e.g. sodium acetate). The concentration of sodium acetate required is found by solving the Henderson–Hasselbalch equation (equation 1.6).

$$pH = pK_a + \log \frac{[SALT]}{[ACID]}$$

$$5.0 = 4.76 + \log\left(\frac{x}{0.1}\right)$$

$x = 0.1738$ M sodium acetate

(d)   The buffer capacity, β, is easily calculated. Suppose we add 0.01 mol of strong alkali (e.g. NaOH). The new pH can be calculated from the Henderson–Hasselbalch equation (1.6).

$$pH = 4.76 + \log \frac{(0.1738 + 0.01)}{0.09}$$

$$pH = 5.07$$

The buffer capacity is defined as the number of moles of strong alkali added divided by change in pH observed.

$$\beta = \frac{0.01}{0.07}$$

$$\beta = 0.14$$

A1.3   The fully protonated form of lysine has the structure shown in Figure 10.1.

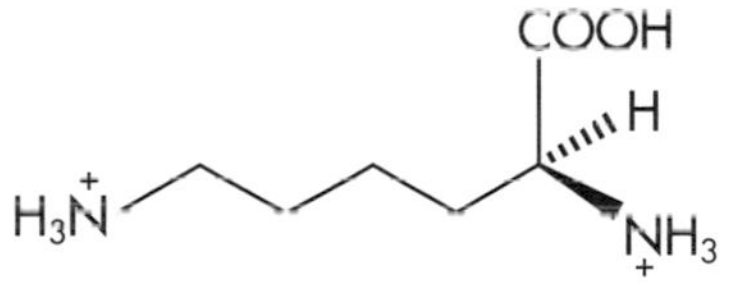

Figure 10.1   The structure of lysine.

The hydrogens ionise in the following order: the first from the carboxy group on the α carbon; the second from the NH_3^+ on the terminal carbon (the ε carbon); and finally the hydrogen from the NH_3^+ on the α carbon. The predominant structure at the pI is the zwitterion, which has the structure shown in Figure 10.2.

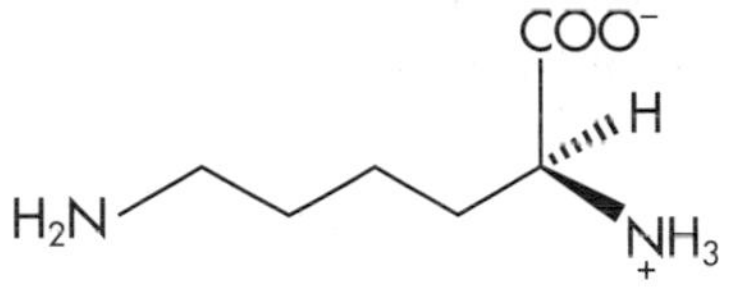

Figure 10.2   The structure of the lysine zwitterion.

A2.1   The true partition coefficient is the partition coefficient for the unionised molecule.

P_{true} is a constant for a given drug and allows comparison of P values for different molecules. The apparent partition coefficient is the partition coefficient measured in the laboratory. If the drug in question ionises, P_{app} will vary with the pH of measurement. This may be measured either by a shake flask method (e.g. using ether and pH 7 buffer) or by chromatography. P_{app} would be measured first and P_{true} calculated using equation (2.2).

$$P_{app} = P \times f_{unionised}$$

The first step is to calculate P_{app} using equation (2.2).

$$P_{app} = P \times f_{unionised}$$

$$P_{app} = 125 \times 0.0156$$

$$P_{app} = 1.950$$

Using equation (2.3),

$$\frac{W_n}{W} = \left(\frac{A}{PS + A}\right)^n$$

$$\frac{W_n}{W} = \left(\frac{4}{(1.95 \times 5 + 4)}\right)^2$$

$$\frac{W_n}{W} = 0.0846$$

The concentration in chloroform is 15.8 μg mL^{-1} in 2 mL and therefore

The amount in chloroform = 31.6 μg

Since the fraction remaining in the aqueous phase is 0.0846,

The fraction extracted = $(1 - 0.0846) = 0.9154$

Therefore, 31.6 μg = 91.54% of total, so

$$\text{Total amount} = \frac{31.6}{0.9154} = 34.52 \ \mu g$$

The initial concentration is given by 34.52 μg in 4 mL, which equals 8.63 μg mL^{-1}. The percentage of drug extracted is obviously $(31.6/34.52) \times 100 = 91.5\%$.

The percentage extracted could be increased by repeating the experiment with dilute mineral acid replacing the buffer. Since the pK_a of sulfamethoxazole is 5.6, carrying out the extraction at a pH of less than 2.6 (drug >99.9% unionised) will allow more of the drug to dissolve in the organic layer.

A2.2   This question is similar to 2.1 above. P_{app} is first calculated from equation (2.2) to give $P_{app} = 1.724$.

The fraction unextracted can be calculated from equation (2.3) and is equal to 0.135.

The weight of drug extracted is given by $0.604 \times 5 = 3.02 \mu g$. The initial amount of drug is found from $3.02/(1 - 0.135) = 3.49 \mu g$ and the original concentration is simply $3.49/5 = 0.698 \mu g\ mL^{-1}$.

The percentage extracted is given by $100(1 - 0.135) = 86.5\%$. This percentage may be increased by carrying out the extraction at high pH so that the basic atenolol is virtually 100% unionised. This will be achieved at a pH of $(9.6 + 3) = 12.6$, or above.

A3.1   Sulfamethoxazole is a sulfonamide derivative and behaves as a weak acid in solution. Trimethoprim contains a diaminopyrimidine group and is therefore a weak base. If a student goes wrong here, the whole question will be wrong and that would be a shame because this is basically an easy separation with more than one correct answer. The principle is to selectively ionise one drug, remove it in the aqueous phase and back extract into fresh organic phase by addition of suitable reagent.

The tablets are crushed, the active ingredients (sulfamethoxazole and trimethoprim) are dissolved in a suitable organic solvent (e.g. toluene or ethyl acetate) and insoluble excipients are removed by filtration. The toluene solution is placed in a separating funnel and hydrochloric acid is added. Addition of acid will ionise the trimethoprim, which will become more water soluble and enter the aqueous (lower) phase. The aqueous phase is removed to a second funnel, whereupon addition of base (e.g. sodium hydroxide solution) will regenerate trimethoprim free base. This can then be back extracted into an organic solvent, removed and dried $(MgSO_4)$, and trimethoprim can be isolated by evaporation of organic solvent. If this extraction is carried out exhaustively, no trimethoprim will remain in the original organic phase, which may be evaporated to yield sulfamethoxazole.

Alternatively, the sulfamethoxazole may be converted to its sodium salt by addition of sodium hydroxide solution. The sulfamethoxazole sodium will be more soluble in the aqueous phase and can be removed as above, acidified with mineral acid (e.g. dilute hydrochloric acid solution) and extracted into fresh orgainc solvent. The organic phase is dried and evaporated as before. This will leave trimethoprim in the original organic layer.

A3.2   The answers are shown in Figure 10.3.

1(a)

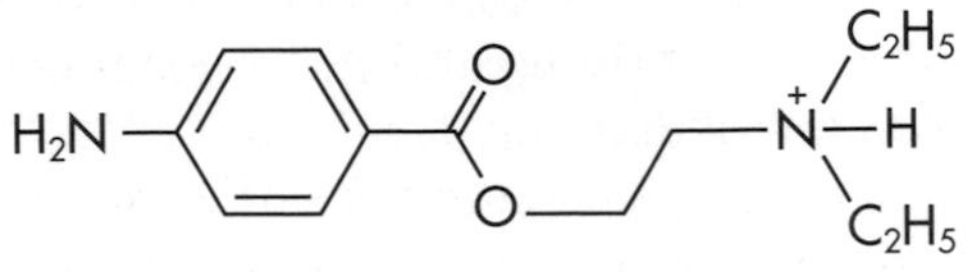

2(c)

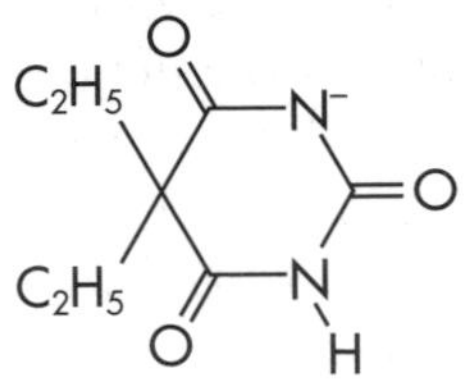

3(c)

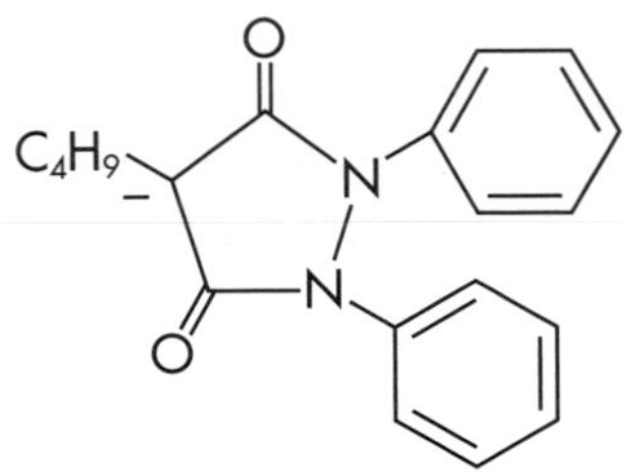

4(a)

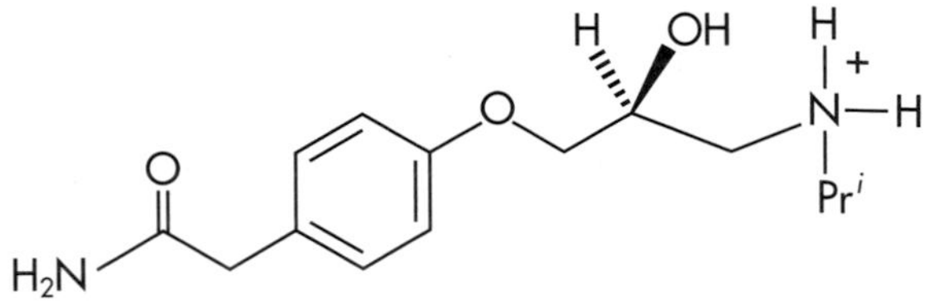

5(e) CH_3CH_2OH

6(c)

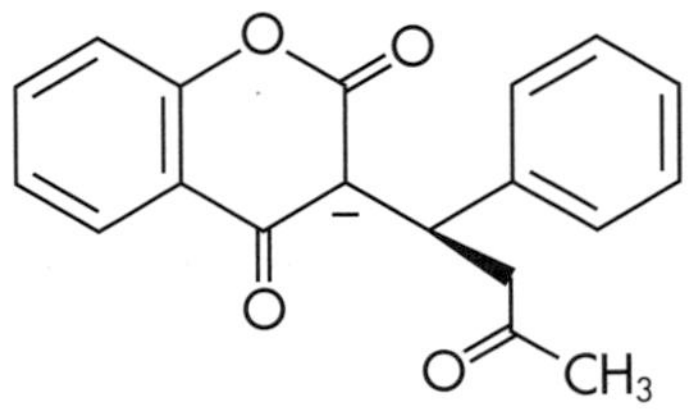

Figure 10.3   Structures of drugs.

A3.3   Nicotine is the addictive alkaloid found in leaves of the tobacco plant (*Nicotiana tabacum* or *N. rustica*). It is a colourless or pale yellow oil that darkens on exposure to air (due to oxidation). Pure nicotine is a deadly poison with an LD_{50} in mice of 0.3 mg kg^{-1} if given intravenously. From the structure shown in Figure 3.26, nicotine is clearly a base with two basic centres. The pyridine nitrogen has a pK_a of 6.16, while the N-methylpyrrolidine has a pK_a of 10.96. This means that only one of the nitrogen atoms is sufficiently basic to ionise at a pH of 7.4, so the structure of nicotine that predominates at the pH of plasma is the mono-cation shown in Figure 10.4. Since the mono-cation predominates at the pH of blood and intracellular fluid, it would be reasonable to assume that this is the form that is active at the receptor. Further evidence for the active form of nicotine is given by considering the natural agonist. The compound the nicotinic receptor is designed to recognise is the neurotransmitter acetylcholine, which, as can be seen from Figure 10.4, is a quaternary ammonium compound. Acetylcholine is ionised at all values of pH and it follows that its receptor will contain negatively charged residues to bind the positive charge. Ionised nicotine is sufficiently similar to acetylcholine to interact with this receptor and exert its toxic action.

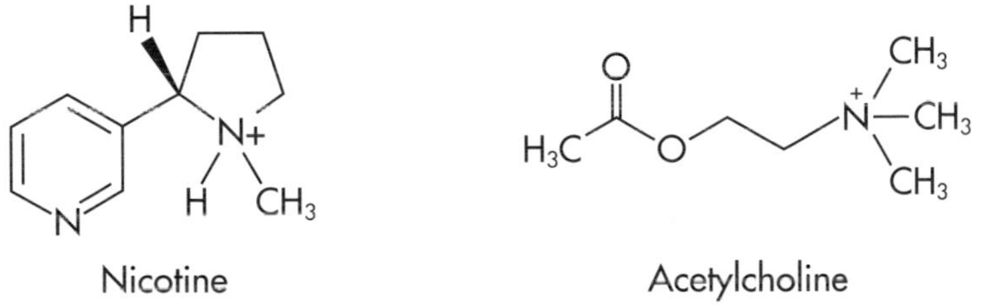

Nicotine   Acetylcholine

Figure 10.4   Structures of nicotine and acetylcholine that predominate at plasma pH.

A4.1   The answers are shown in Figure 10.5. Incidentally, dimercaprol is also known as British Anti Lewisite (or BAL) and was originally developed as an antidote to the chemical warfare agent Lewisite, an arsenic derivative.

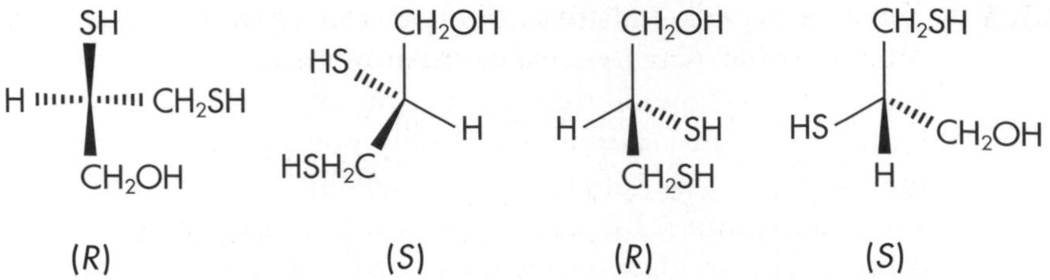

Figure 10.5   Representations of dimercaprol.

A4.2   The answers are shown in Figure 10.6.

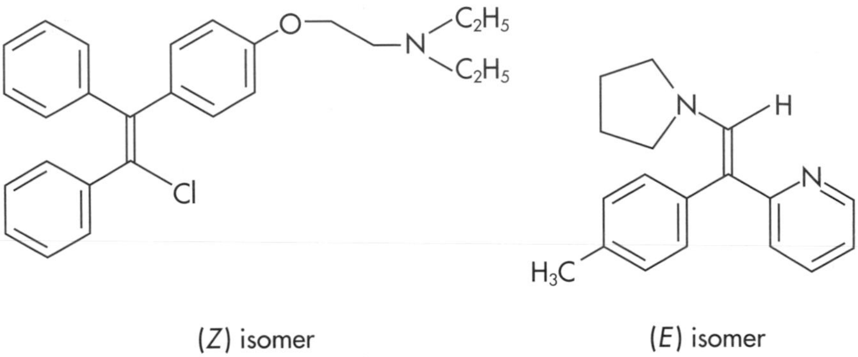

(Z) isomer   (E) isomer

Figure 10.6   The designation of geometrical isomers.

A4.3   Naloxone hydrochloride is (5R, 14S).

Around the 5-position, the oxygen of the epoxide takes priority 1, the carbonyl group is 2, and the rest of the molecule is 3. With the hydrogen projecting out of the page, the direction of priority would be O, C=O, ring, which would be (S). However, when viewed from the side opposite the group with lowest priority, the designation must be (R).

The situation at the 14-position is a little more complicated. Priority 1 goes to the OH, priority 2 to the carbon attached to the basic nitrogen, priority 3 to the carbon in the 13-position and priority 4 to the carbon in the 8-position. It follows that priorities 1, 2, 3 lie anticlockwise and therefore the designation is (S).

A5.1   There is actually more than one correct answer to this question. Possible metabolic transformations are:

- *Aliphatic hydroxylation* – meprobamate
- *Oxidative N-dealkylation* – pethidine (or procaine)
- *Hydrolysis* – procaine (or pethidine)
- *Aromatic hydroxylation* – phenylbutazone (or pethidine)
- *Oxidative O-dealkylation* – phenacetin

The structures of the metabolites are shown in Figure 10.7.

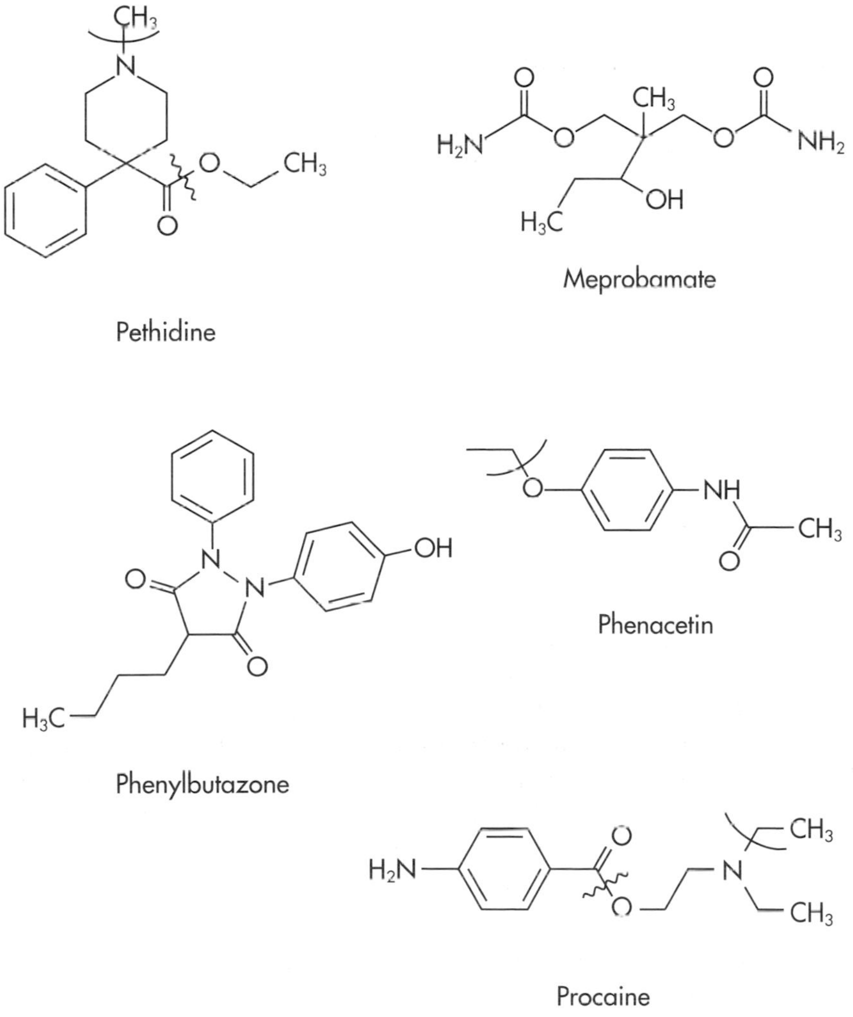

Pethidine

Meprobamate

Phenylbutazone

Phenacetin

Procaine

Figure 10.7   The structures of drug metabolites.

A5.2   Phase 1 reactions are sometimes described as 'non-synthetic' reactions and involve chemical modification of functional groups in the drug molecule (hydrolysis, oxidation, etc.). Polar groups are introduced, or existing polar functional groups are unmasked. The Phase 1 derivative is usually more water soluble (hydrophilic) than the parent drug. A Phase 2 (or 'synthetic') derivative usually involves covalent bond formation to yield a water-soluble conjugate (e.g. glucuronide, sulfate). Phase 2 reactions may occur on the parent drug or on the product of a Phase 1 metabolic conversion.

A6.1   (a)   Back titrations are used where the forward reaction is slow or does not proceed 100% to the right-hand side.

(b)
$$Li_2CO_3 + 2HCl \rightarrow 2LiCl + H_2O + CO_2$$
$$2HCl + 2NaOH \rightarrow 2NaCl + 2H_2O$$

Therefore, since the relative molecular mass of Li_2CO_3 is 73.9,

$$73.9 \text{ g } Li_2CO_3 \equiv 2000 \text{ mL 1 M NaOH}$$
$$0.03695 \text{ g } Li_2CO_3 \equiv 1 \text{ mL 1 M NaOH}$$

(c)   (i)   100.1% w/w.
   (ii)   An answer >100% suggests a basic impurity, which is using up titrant in the same way as the sample; probably another metal carbonate.
   (iii)   A suitable indicator would be methyl orange. Dissolved carbon dioxide in the sample may ionise to produce an acidic solution; therefore an indicator that changes on the acid side of neutrality is required.

A6.2   (a)   This technique is a non-aqueous titration, which is used for the assay of compounds that are insufficiently acidic or basic to provide a sharp end point in aqueous solution. Precautions to be observed are to carry out the assay in totally anhydrous conditions. This means that all glassware, apparatus and solutions used should be dry.

(b)   The solution of perchloric acid should be standardised using a primary standard, i.e. a compound that can be obtained in a very high level of purity. In the case of perchloric acid, either benzoic acid or potassium hydrogen phthalate would be suitable.

(c) The equivalent relationship is that 1 mL of 0.1 M $HClO_4$ is equivalent to 0.02112 g of methyldopa, which gives a purity of the sample of 99.6%.

A6.3 (a) This is a REDOX (oxidation–reduction) titration. The cerium *gains an electron* and is *reduced*, while the ascorbic acid *loses two electrons* and is *oxidised*.

(b) The equivalent relationship is 1 mL of 0.1 M ACS ≡ 0.008806 g ascorbic acid. The weight of ascorbic acid in the sample is 0.1676 g. The number of tablets assayed is 3.1298. The content of ascorbic acid in a tablet of average weight is 0.0535 g and the percentage stated amount is 107.1%.

(c) The pK_a values are assigned to the ene-diol system as shown in Figure 10.8. The huge discrepancy in acidity is due to delocalisation of the negative charge formed on the first ionisation and subsequent hydrogen bonded stabilisation of the mono-anion. Subsequent ionisation results in loss of this stabilising effect and is therefore unfavourable.

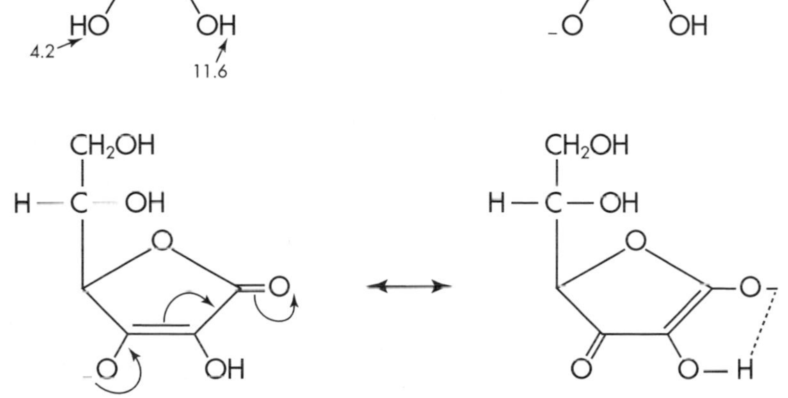

Figure 10.8 Resonance effects of ascorbic acid.

It is important to avoid confusion between the processes of *ionisation* and *oxidation*. When ascorbic acid ionises, the hydrogen leaves as an *ion* (H⁺) and its electron remains on the molecule to form an anion, whereas when the molecule is oxidised the hydrogen leaves along with its electron to give a diketone. These two processes are quite different and ascorbic acid is a good molecule to demonstrate the difference.

A7.1 (a) All unsaturated regions of the molecule, i.e. both benzene rings plus C=C and C=O double bonds. This region is called the chromophore.

(b) The major assumption is that the Beer–Lambert law applies to this assay. Other assumptions are that no tablet excipients absorb at 284 nm, and that the extraction procedure is 100% effective.

(c) Content of $C_{16}H_{13}ClN_2O$ in a tablet of average weight is 4.73 mg; percentage stated amount is 94.7%.

(d) Diazepam could be assayed by a number of techniques, including non-aqueous titration, $AgNO_3$ titration, gravimetric assay, etc.

A7.2 (a) The content of mepyramine in a tablet of average weight is 52.69 mg and the percentage stated amount is 105.4%.

(b) The sample is centrifuged to remove insoluble tablet excipients.

(c) Mepyramine is basic (tertiary amine $pK_a = 8.9$); therefore, hydrochloric acid is used to ensure that all the mepyramine is converted to the water-soluble hydrochloride salt. This will allow all the mepyramine to be extracted from the crushed tablet matrix.

(d) A blank solution is everything except the sample. Therefore, the blank would have to be prepared exactly as stated for the test, but with the sample omitted.

A8.1 (a) The benzylic positions and, in particular, the phenol are likely to undergo oxidation on storage (Figure 10.9).

(b) The groups susceptible to hydrolysis are the amide, the cyclic ester (a lactone), the glycoside and the carbamate (Figure 10.9).

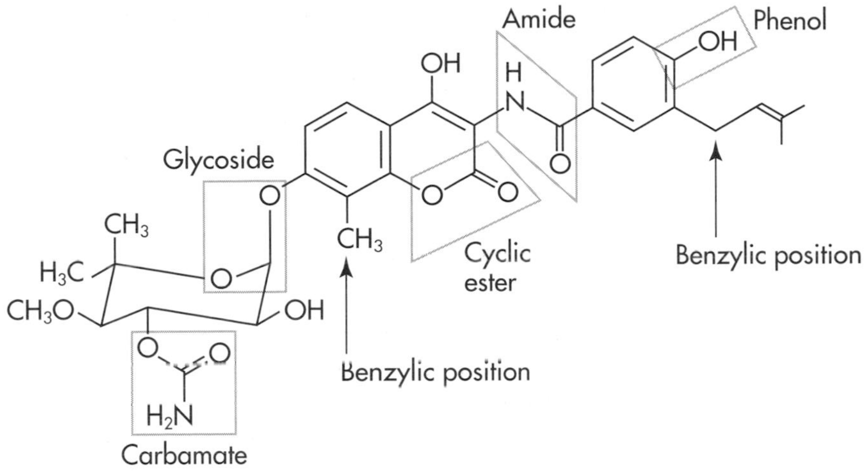

Figure 10.9 The structure of novobiocin.

(c) Novobiocin should be stored in an airtight container and protected from light.

(d) The drug must be water soluble when administered in an infusion. This is achieved by forming the sodium salt of novobiocin. As this is the salt of a weak acid and a strong base, aqueous solutions are alkaline by partial hydrolysis (revise Chapter 1 if you do not follow this!). When the drug is added to a 5% Dextrose Infusion (pH 3.5–6.5), the pH of the solution is sufficiently low to precipitate the water-insoluble free acid of novobiocin from solution of the salt, turning the solution cloudy. If this precipitation occurs in the infusion bag, an expensive medicine is ruined. If the precipitation occurs in the vein of a seriously ill patient, the consequences could be catastrophic (to the pharmacist who did not recognise the incompatibility as well as to the unfortunate patient).

A8.2 (a) Penicillins are unstable in aqueous solution, and therefore cannot be supplied in liquid form. This is due to aqueous hydrolysis of the strained β-lactam ring. The mechanism is shown in Figure 10.10.

(b) The catechol OH groups of adrenaline (epinephrine) undergo oxidation to adrenochrome (see Figure 10.11) red pigment, which imparts a pink colour to adrenaline

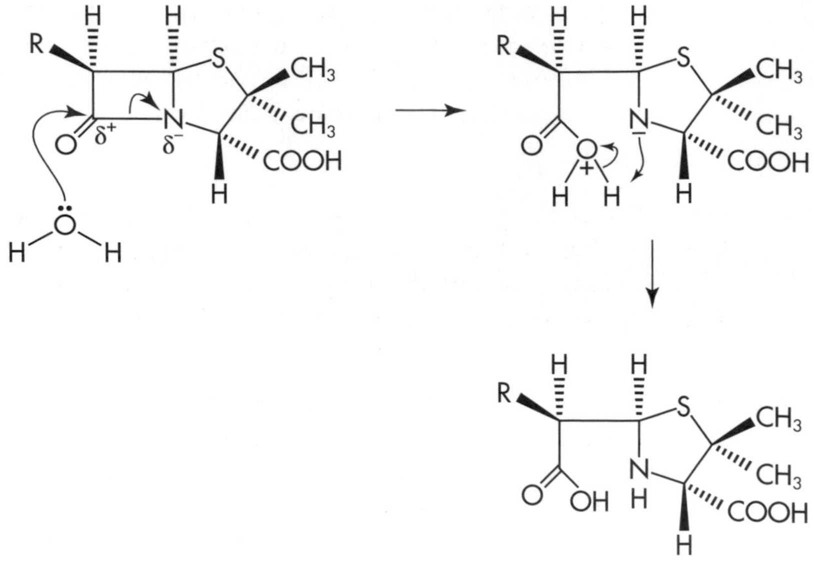

Figure 10.10 The mechanism of penicillin hydrolysis.

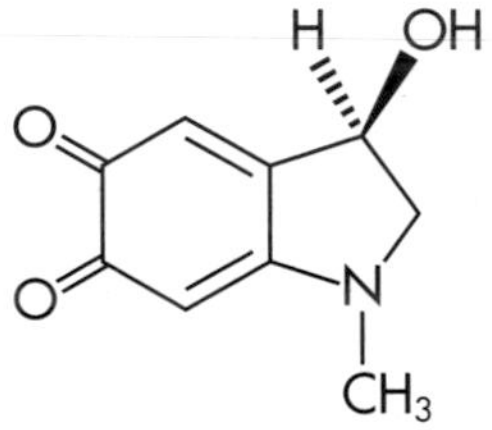

Figure 10.11 The structure of adrenochrome.

solutions. Adrenochrome may be further oxidised to melanin, the dark pigment of human skin, hair, etc.

(c) Aspirin (or acetylsalicylic acid) is an ester and is easily hydrolysed to yield salicylic and acetic acids. The latter possesses a strong vinegar-like odour. This process can occur even when aspirin is present in tablet form. The mechanism is similar to the hydrolysis of penicillin shown above.

(d) Angiotensin II is an octapeptide composed of eight amino acids joined to each other by peptide bonds. Peptidase enzymes present in the body can hydrolyse these bonds to liberate free amino acids. It is often the case that potent biological molecules (e.g. hormones such as adrenaline, or neurotransmitters such as acetylcholine) are quickly broken down either chemically or by enzymes. This rapidly terminates the biological activity.

A9.1 For a first-order process, $\ln(a - x) = \ln a - kt$ and a plot of $\ln(a - x)$ vs t should give a straight line graph with slope equal to $-k$. This graph was plotted and a slope of -0.351 was obtained. Thus, negative slope $= -k$ and hence $k = 0.351$ day^{-1}.

A9.2 (a) For a first-order process, $\ln(a - x) = \ln a - kt$ and a plot of $\ln(a - x)$ vs t should give a straight line graph with slope equal to $-k$. This graph was plotted and a slope of -0.00412 was obtained. Thus, negative slope equals $-k$ and hence $k = 0.00412$ s^{-1}. The fact that this equation yields a straight line confirms the rate is first order with respect to peroxide.

(b) Using the linear form of the Arrhenius equation,

$$\ln k = \ln A - \frac{E}{R} \times \frac{1}{T}$$

A plot of $\ln k$ vs $1/T$ will yield a graph of slope $-E/R$, from which E, the activation energy, may be calculated (units are J mol^{-1} or kJ mol^{-1}).

To determine the frequency factor, a pair of values of $\ln k$ and $1/T$ are chosen, the above graph is plotted and the intercept with the vertical axis is determined. This is $\ln A$, from which A, the frequency factor, is found. The units of A are the same as for k, i.e. s^{-1}.

Index

Drug names are in **bold** type.

Page numbers in *italic* refer to figures.